BIG & BOLD:

Strength Training for the Plus-Size Woman

Morit Summers, CPT

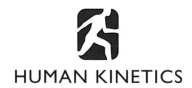

HUMAN KINETICS

Library of Congress Cataloging-in-Publication Data

Names: Summers, Morit, 1986- author.
Title: Big & bold : strength training for the plus-size woman / Morit
  Summers.
Other titles: Big and bold
Description: Champaign, IL : Human Kinetics, [2022]
Identifiers: LCCN 2021010203 (print) | LCCN 2021010204 (ebook) | ISBN
  9781718200050 (paperback) | ISBN 9781718200067 (epub) | ISBN
  9781718200074 (pdf)
Subjects: LCSH: Physical fitness for women. | Overweight women. |
  Overweight women--Health and hygiene. | Weight training for women.
Classification: LCC GV482 .S86 2022 (print) | LCC GV482 (ebook) | DDC
  613.7/045--dc23
LC record available at https://lccn.loc.gov/2021010203
LC ebook record available at https://lccn.loc.gov/2021010204

ISBN: 978-1-7182-0005-0 (print)

This publication is written and published to provide accurate and authoritative information relevant to the subject matter presented. It is published and sold with the understanding that the author and publisher are not engaged in rendering legal, medical, or other professional services by reason of their authorship or publication of this work. If medical or other expert assistance is required, the services of a competent professional person should be sought.

The web addresses cited in this text were current as of December 2020, unless otherwise noted.

Senior Acquisitions Editor: Michelle Maloney; **Senior Developmental Editor:** Cynthia McEntire; **Managing Editor:** Hannah Werner; **Copyeditor:** E before I Editing; **Permissions Manager:** Dalene Reeder; **Senior Graphic Designer:** Joe Buck; **Cover Designer:** Keri Evans; **Cover Design Specialist:** Susan Rothermel Allen; **Photograph (cover):** Anthony Cunanan / Human Kinetics, Inc.; **Photographs (interior):** Anthony Cunanan; **Photo Production Specialist:** Amy M. Rose; **Photo Production Manager:** Jason Allen; **Senior Art Manager:** Kelly Hendren; **Illustrations:** © Human Kinetics; **Printer:** Versa Press

We thank FORM Fitness Brooklyn in Brooklyn, New York, for assistance in providing the location for the photo shoots for this book.

Human Kinetics books are available at special discounts for bulk purchase. Special editions or book excerpts can also be created to specification. For details, contact the Special Sales Manager at Human Kinetics.

Printed in the United States of America   10 9 8 7 6 5 4 3 2 1

The paper in this book is certified under a sustainable forestry program.

Human Kinetics
1607 N. Market Street
Champaign, IL 61820
USA

United States and International
Website: **US.HumanKinetics.com**
Email: info@hkusa.com
Phone: 1-800-747-4457

Canada
Website: **Canada.HumanKinetics.com**
Email: info@hkcanada.com

E8150

Tell us what you think!
Human Kinetics would love to hear what we can do to improve the customer experience. Use this QR code to take our brief survey.

*To all my big and bold women
who not only lift weights, but
also lift those around them each
and every day.*

CONTENTS

Part I   Set for Success

Chapter 1   Find Your Why 3

Strength training is not just about our physical being—it's also about our mental being. Learn about the different types of strength, their importance, and ways to work toward a stronger body and mind.

Chapter 2   Prepare to Move 15

Start your strength training journey. There is so much to understand when starting a fitness journey. Learn about setting goals, setting your workout schedule, and determining what you need to take that first step.

Part II   Get Moving

Chapter 3   Squat and Hinge 37

Discover the specific movements you will use on this journey. Learn to perform the squat, deadlift, and many other lower-body exercises. Because not everyone is at the same point in their journey, there are variations of each exercise—for beginners through advanced lifters—so you can incorporate the movement that feels the most appropriate for you.

Chapter 4   Push and Pull 69

Perfect the upper-body exercises you will use during your journey. All movements are presented with many variations and options so you can make the movements work for you. Women sometimes have a harder time developing upper-body strength; we will discuss this and learn to use the whole body to push and get stronger.

Chapter 5   Anti-Rotation, Loaded Carry, and Rotation 105

Let's move on to the core, an incredibly important part of strength. Learn to perform loaded carries, rotation movements, and anti-rotation movements. It is possible to work the core without getting on the ground; we will discuss different options.

Part III Make a Plan

Chapter 6 Create Your Workout

Learn to put together a workout. Find the right options for you to program a workout routine that meets your needs. What programming methods make the most sense for you, and why? You will learn all about repetitions, sets, load, and rest periods and all the ways to progress your workouts.

Chapter 7 Sample Workouts

There are many ways to get strong. Find sample workouts that provide options for beginner, intermediate, and advanced lifters. See what a workout plan looks like.

Chapter 8 Take Action

Now that you have all the tools in your toolbox, let's talk about what it takes to make your workouts happen. Start slow: Two workouts a week can increase to three, and so on. Clarify your thoughts and get started on this journey.

EXERCISE FINDER

ANTI-ROTATION, LOADED CARRY, AND ROTATION

WARM UP

SAMPLE WORKOUTS

SERIES PREFACE

I'm going to say it: *Fitness* is a loaded word.

My Amazonian body won me gold ribbons, crossed the finish line first in races, was awarded a coveted athletic scholarship to Syracuse, and led what began as a personal passion into a global movement for inclusive beauty decades ago.

For me, being fit is a source of joy and accomplishment. It's in my blood. I get out a few times each week and every weekend to smell the air and put miles under my feet. The more time I'm in nature during every season, the happier I am.

My commitment to living a fit lifestyle is nonnegotiable, even if I don't fit the cultural ideal of what healthy or fit looks like. But millions of women face judgment, a disparaging word, or a disapproving glance, especially when a gleeful, confident, and curvy bod announces her triathlon goals or athletic accomplishment on an IG feed or—God forbid—skips by in real time.

It seriously makes me wonder: Why do happy, fit, and curvy people piss so many off, and why is *fit* a term for a select few?

No, my sweaty, joyous souls; fitness includes all body shapes, ages, and sizes! The Cooper Institute in Dallas tapped into this years ago when their data and research reflected an array of body types, not just the very thin, that could (and do) achieve fitness. Being fit is something all of us can set as a goal and attain, regardless of size.

Why on earth should only a few folks be able to claim a fit and healthy life? We all come in various shapes and sizes—be it tall and angular, naturally muscular, or naturally curvier. When we add our skeletal structures for each body type (i.e., XS, S, M, L, XL, XXL, XXXL), there's a bouquet of human expression going on that includes those embracing a fit lifestyle. When I break down who we are in this way, it makes sense to me and allows me to be who I am and not try to be what I'm not. Fitness is a journey open and available to all shapes and sizes (and ages)!

But how do we hold on to this inclusive mindset?

First, your purse is your power tool. Ignore marketing designed to motivate a purchase and make companies a lot of money. Second, don't buy into false beliefs that fitness, beauty, and success are an exclusive membership for the select few. It's time to get off the never-ending hamster wheel fueled by self-defeating diets and the mindset of "fitting in" and ask yourself, "For what?"

We're all in this together for goodness' sake, and I've got a news flash—this is *so* not a size thing; it's a women's rights issue. I beg you: Get off that train to nowhere *now* and allow yourself to be totally absorbed in the magic within the pages of this book. They will set you free from body bashing, comparisons, and put-downs and set you in a new direction of self-discovery that you never thought possible. All it takes is one step, then another, then another, and you're off enjoying *your* fitness journey.

Start by creating your own story. Be your own sweaty badass babe rocking life, no matter what. Own it and claim *you*! Once you drop the mic on limiting beliefs, others will wonder where all your fabulousness is coming from and become curious about the miracles being performed in your life. Start; you'll see. Dance, swim, glide, ride, walk, run, and sway; allow various forms of movement to flow through you as your new self-expression.

Above all, by engaging in our own fitness routines for the sheer joy of play as if our lives depend on it, we unleash our very own superpower to be fit under our terms, regardless of our size. Our glorious, magnificent, and powerful body pumps blood every day without being told to do so and allows us to live this incredible life. Honor it by slowing down to listen to it. Once we become our own body's bodyguard, the stars align and a path is cleared to a life *we* get to choose.

Fitness is by no means a race to the fittest; it's a lifestyle. With intention. A life committed to joy, wellness, and getting a kick out of being fit. I'm excited for you. An empowering new frame of mind around fitness is awaiting you here.

In joy,
xo
Emme
#playsweatwin

PREFACE

This book is for any woman who wants to become the best version of herself. It's for the woman who wants to learn how to get stronger but is intimidated by the gym or can't afford a personal trainer. If you don't know where to begin, this book will help! The gym can be an intimidating place, but I didn't let that get in my way, and I want to help other women learn to be less intimidated too.

I've been called fat my entire life. I have been doubted and bullied every step of the way. I have happy memories just like the next person, but the memories that stick out the most are the ones of friends looking at me and saying things like "Wow, you got fat." I was bullied on teams and school buses. Coaches told me that I could sit the mile out instead of pushing me to at least try or to walk it. I felt incapable and thought that I wasn't good enough. My parents took me to the doctor multiple times to see if there was something wrong with me that caused me to weigh more than my peers. I was forced to play sports, which left me feeling defeated. All I wanted was to fit in, but no one else was fat. Even if there were other big kids, I didn't even notice anything about what they were going through because I was worried about myself—worried all the time about what everyone else thought about me. I wanted to be like all the skinny girls, the girls who the boys liked.

I was constantly embarrassed in gym class and really wanted to lose weight. Finally at age 14, my parents paid for me to work with a personal trainer at the local gym, which I'm grateful for every day. Walking in the gym that day changed my life. My trainer changed my life. We didn't work together for very long, but the impact was huge. I've worked out in gyms ever since, and I have made it my mission to try to change the lives of other women the way my trainer did for me. Not only did she get me moving, but she made me love working out, and she made me realize for the first time that I was capable; I could do anything I put my mind to.

My journey in fitness has changed dramatically. It went from trying to lose weight as the ultimate goal to realizing that I am capable of so much more. I always knew that I wanted to be a personal trainer because I wanted to help change people's lives, but I also had a selfish reason for pursuing this profession. I wanted to be able to work out and be surrounded by other people who liked to work out and be healthy like me. Yet doing so had a negative effect for a long time. In trying to keep up with my peers and doing anything to lose weight, I was not always successful, so I felt really discouraged at times. My managers at work made me feel that I wouldn't succeed because I was fat—even though I was proving them wrong when I became the top personal trainer at a huge company. I did that by using my knowledge of fitness to attract clients. Once they knew I could give them a good workout and that I cared about their well-being, they didn't see the "fat" me; they saw the smart, professional me.

Even though professionally I was a success, I still felt like I didn't fit in. I wanted to lose weight and look like the other trainers. I had been in the gym and lifting weights since age 14, but it wasn't until I was about 27 years old that I truly understood what lifting weights could mean. I fell into CrossFit and powerlifting. Besides the fact that I loved the community, I realized that there was a way for me to see progress besides a number on the scale. There was a way for me to feel mentally strong and to prove everyone wrong. Even with all the education I had, it wasn't until CrossFit and powerlifting that I realized I could measure goals outside of my weight on the scale; I could measure my workouts, the weights I was able to lift, how fast I was able to move. All of these were concepts I always knew but they never really registered.

Suddenly my passion for fitness was bigger and better than ever. My motivation skyrocketed and I wanted to get stronger and stronger. I have since competed in CrossFit, Olympic weightlifting, and powerlifting competitions. I've studied and implemented more effective strength training protocols. In some ways, I wish I had realized all this much earlier in my fitness and professional career. It would have helped me avoid a lot of hurt and discouragement. But my path to fitness helps me understand where my current clients and followers are coming from and the challenges they face every day. It is hard to want to work out if you're always struggling to lose weight or to fit in or to do what everyone else expects you to do or to do what doctors believe is best for you. You are in charge of your strength and your level of effort. You can cut out all those years of discouragement and start working on being more confident and stronger now. I'm still "overweight," but I'm super strong and I am capable, and I can help you be the same!

ACKNOWLEDGMENTS

I never, even in my wildest dreams, thought that I would ever write a book. It has always been my dream—and the core goal of my decision to pursue a career in fitness—to help and make a difference for people, even if only in a small way. I am grateful for the opportunity I have been given to write this book and to be able to reach people in a way I didn't think possible for me before. I want to thank the whole team at Human Kinetics for working so hard on this project with me over the last year; special thanks to Michelle, Cynthia, Doug, Amy, Joe, Jason, Heidi, and Keri for helping me turn my thoughts and ideas into this incredible book. Anthony, thank you for making the images come alive. Tiffany and Tina, thank you for showing us how to be big and bold.

I also want to say thank you to everyone in my life who helped me get to this point. Francine, my best friend and business partner, thank you for never letting me forget that I am capable of greatness. Rose, my friend I can't get rid of, but really who can't get rid of me, my younger sister (who acts like she's my older sister), and basically my life manager, thank you for always supporting me and helping me reach my goals. Jowan, thank you for being you, for always being positive and bright and solid as a rock. To all my clients, without you putting your trust in me, and sticking with me, I wouldn't be where I am today. To my gigantic family and all my friends, and the strong women who raised me and grew up with me, I love you and thank you. I especially want to thank my Instagram community for shaping the last few years of my life and my businesses. The support I received from you is what gave me the courage to take major steps like open FORM Fitness Brooklyn and to write this book. It's an incredible thing knowing that people want to hear what you have to say.

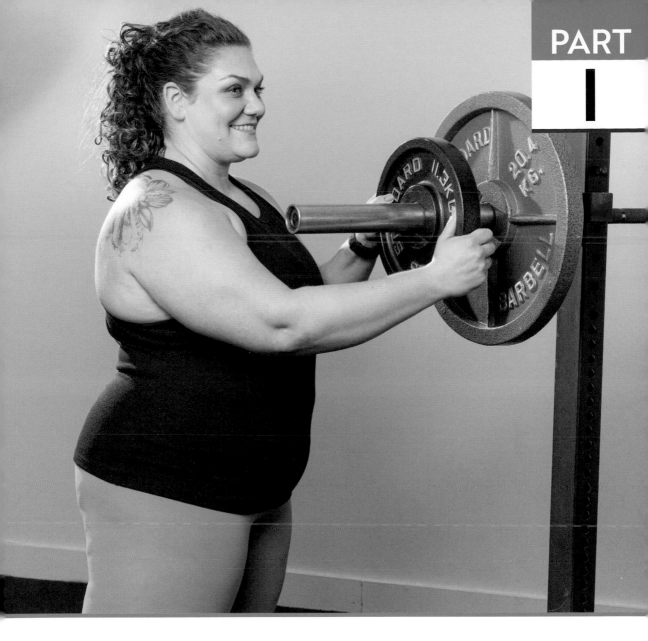

Set for Success

CHAPTER 1

FIND YOUR WHY

We've all been there: standing next to our seat upon boarding the airplane, desperate to get a suitcase in the overhead bin. Or maybe you're out and about with your kids, trying to carry the stroller up a flight of stairs. Whatever the action may be, the idea is the same: Everyday life requires that we be capable and strong. We usually don't give a second thought to the movements and actions our days ask of us. We carry the laundry from the basement all the way upstairs; it's not a big deal. Or is it? Strength is something we started gaining from birth. But strength is not something that simply sticks around. We have to work hard and put in the repetitions for our muscles to grow and our bodies to get stronger.

Strength training can take different forms. When people talk about strength training, they're usually referring to lifting weights. That's one form of building strength, and in this book, I'm going to help prepare you for that. But I am also going to guide you through some of the mental components of strength training.

OUR VERY FIRST LEARNED MOVEMENTS

First, let's talk about strength in its purest form: the mastery of bodyweight movements. Every morning, the first thing we do after we get out of bed is head to the bathroom. You sit down, and then you stand again. Let's rephrase that: The first activity you do every day is a squat, which is one of the most fundamental movements a human can do.

From the time we were born, we started getting stronger. Without thinking about it, we learned to lift our giant baby heads. Then we learned to roll over, sit up, crawl, stand, and walk. For most of us, these things happened naturally, but you did have to work for it. If you have kids, you have watched your children try to do something over and over and over again, until—bam!—they got it. If you don't have kids, ask your parents. You didn't come out of the womb walking. You worked toward it. You did so many repetitions to gain the strength to hold your own head up. It took repetitions to roll over, to lift yourself up onto your knees, to pull yourself up on your feet, and then eventually to take a step, just to fall on your butt again. You did this over and over until you were strong enough to walk. You walked right into school—and started to lose all that strength that you had worked so hard for. You sat down. Take a moment to think about how little you actually move in a day. We sit to eat meals, sit to watch TV, and lie down to go to bed. Many of us sit during work. Think about how much time you are fighting against your own body to keep yourself strong. As I'm writing this, I'm noticing how long I have been sitting and I'm thinking, "Man, I really need to stand up soon."

We have learned movement patterns that cause our movements to be done by instinct. These patterns are our muscles in use. Unfortunately, these movement patterns can fade. You continue to know how to walk unless something happens to you that prohibits you from doing so. However, for most of us, these patterns won't be as strong since we sit all day. It's estimated that, without some form of movement or exercise, muscular endurance starts fading after two weeks and overall muscular strength after about a month. Our bodies need muscle to function properly; our bodies need muscle just to get us to stand up.

PRESIDENTIAL FITNESS TESTING (A.K.A. THE THING WE'D ALL LIKE TO FORGET)

Who remembers gym class? If you were anything like me, you have tried hard to make those memories go away. Personally, I hated gym class (also called physical education). I hated being the only kid who couldn't run in circles around the gym without being lapped multiple times and feeling totally incapable and out of shape. Right now I can picture the coach saying, "Okay, warm up," and expect us to run laps around the gym. To this day, you could tell me to run laps in circles and I revert to my former self, out of breath and anxious about it. Gym made me feel less than, like I couldn't keep up. Then there was the Presidential Physical Fitness Test: push-ups, sit-ups, flexibility, and running. Clear as day, I remember hearing the coaches say, "If you don't hit the standards, you will fail gym." Who fails gym class? How is that motivating?

Here's a breakdown of what the Presidential Physical Fitness Test consisted of, for those lucky enough to have never encountered it. The activities were each supposed to be completed within a certain time limit. The test consisted of five activities:

1. Sit-ups (or crunches) to measure abdominal muscle tone and core strength. Kids performed sit-ups for one minute. A 17-year-old boy was expected to perform 55 and a girl 44.
2. A one-mile run to test aerobic fitness. For older students, the goals were 6 minutes, 6 seconds for boys and 8 minutes, 17 seconds for girls.
3. Pull-ups or right-angle push-ups, as many as possible without stopping, to measure upper-body strength. At 17, a boy had to do 13 pull-ups or 53 push-ups; girls had to do 1 pull-up or 23 push-ups.

4. Shuttle run to measure speed and agility. The student ran 30 feet, picked up a block, ran back and placed the block down, picked up a second block, and ran 30 feet back to place the block down. Boys and girls in the oldest group had to complete the test in 8.7 and 10 seconds, respectively.

5. V-sit reaches to show the flexibility of the muscles in the spine and back of the legs. Students sat on the floor and reached between their legs. The goals were to reach more than 7 inches for 17-year-old boys and more than 8 inches for 17-year-old girls.

What I have come to learn, years after the trauma from the fitness test and gym, is that not everyone has to do the same thing to be healthy. Not everyone is a runner, not everyone is super flexible, and not everyone is super strong. Each year, I would try my best at the sit-ups (my best event; still is), the sit and reach, the push-ups, and then when it came to the run, I wanted to run home and cry—yes, run home. Instead of helping or giving positive feedback on the other events, my coaches acted as though I never even tried, as though I weren't like the rest of my peers.

We need to find some type of activity that we enjoy and want to keep doing. I got lucky, in a weird way. When I couldn't finish the mile in time, I was mortified and discouraged, but it made me want to try harder. Because I wanted to be like the other kids and fit in, I wanted to be able to run the mile and pass gym. To achieve that goal, I trained hard! I was at the gym every day after school practicing on the treadmill. Yes, I made it happen, but as soon as that test was done, I stopped running—and you can guess what went away immediately: my ability and desire to run. What didn't disappear was the eagerness to fit in. I still wanted to lose weight, so I lifted weights and worked out. Even though I didn't love gym class, I loved the gym! I could do it all by myself. There was no judgment from my peers. I realized that while running and sports weren't for me, weights were. We have to find the thing we love, or at least tolerate. Unfortunately, it took me a long time to realize that lifting wasn't about losing weight. It was about lifting, it was about feeling accomplished, it was about being committed, and it was about feeling and being strong.

STRENGTH DEFINED

Strength, simply put, is the state of being strong. Strength can be how much you lift, it can be how hard you work, and most of the time it is both put together. Strength in the world of fitness is how much you can lift. True strength, in fitness, is how much weight you can lift at one time. Most people never actually test their true strength. For most of us, strength is finding our most capable body. Strength is just the state of being strong. What I found was that the more I lifted weights, the stronger I became—yes, physically, but also mentally. I figured out who I was, and I realized that it was okay to hate running. I realized I could be as healthy as people I knew and was comparing myself to. Now I love it so much I'm writing a book about it. Okay, you get it. I love strength training. I'm hoping you will, too, after I break down all things strength.

Strength has so many benefits. Here's a list of a few benefits of strength training. With as little as two times a week you really can see change.

- Develop strong bones. By stressing your bones, strength training can increase bone density and reduce the risk of osteoporosis.
- Manage your weight. Strength training can help you manage or lose weight, and it can increase your metabolism to help you burn more calories. Remember that the number on the scale doesn't mean much, but 200 pounds of fat is very different from 200 pounds of muscle.
- Enhance your quality of life. Strength training may enhance your quality of life and improve your ability to do everyday activities. Building muscle also can contribute to better balance and may reduce your risk of falls. This can help you maintain independence as you age.
- Manage chronic conditions. Strength training can reduce the signs and symptoms of chronic conditions such as arthritis, back pain, heart disease, depression, and diabetes.
- Sharpen your thinking skills. Some research suggests that regular strength training and aerobic exercise may help improve thinking and learning skills for older adults (Mayo Clinic. 2019. "Strength Training: Get Stronger, Leaner, Healthier." February 23, 2019. www.mayoclinic.org/healthy-lifestyle/fitness/in-depth/strength-training/art-20046670.).

I live in New York City, and every day I see mothers with babies in strollers getting off the subway and staring up the staircase. Most don't look around at other people to ask for help; most people don't want to admit when they need help. I'm going to be the first to tell you that if you need to use your arms to get off a chair, it's time to get some help. I'm here to help you, and this book is going to guide you toward a stronger body. Trust me when I tell you that we all have the ability to live a strong, healthy life. That mother is absolutely entitled to need help. That stroller, diaper bag, and baby, collectively, probably weigh more than 60 pounds—not to mention it all comes together in a very awkward shape and size. However, wouldn't it be cool if you were the friend everyone called when they needed help carrying the new piano up the stairs? Maybe that's excessive, and whether you could actually do it or not doesn't matter. In my mind, I'm super strong, I'm capable of anything. Even when I try and fail at something, I still tried.

PERFECT IS FAKE

We put too much pressure on ourselves. Often, the reason people fail is expectations. We want to start a new fitness routine and decided that we have to go to the gym five times a week and can eat only grilled chicken and broccoli. If all the really fit people on the magazine covers and in all of the ads are doing it that way, then it must work. What we forget is that it takes time to make change. I'm also a firm believer that if you want to have a cookie, you should have a cookie—but broccoli is good too. We have to remind ourselves "the pyramids weren't built in a day." As humans, we are growing and learning constantly, but we must allow ourselves time to grow. We aren't perfect—perfect is fake. Perfect isn't realistic. As a plus-size trainer I can truly speak to this. Many people don't respect me as a coach and a trainer because of my size. How can I know what I'm talking about since I'm still fat? I have been in a gym since the age of 14. I went to school and studied exercise science and kinesiology. I have been training people for 14 years. Here is what I know: We don't all have the same goals. We are taught to believe that life will only be awesome, and we will only be healthy, if we look a certain way. We don't all want to look like the model on the cover of *Fitness* magazine; we are told that this is what we want to look like. I'm here to tell you that people can believe what they want, but we can prove them wrong. I have worked with hundreds of clients, and generally during an initial meeting the goals are all similar. "I want to lose weight," "I want to be stronger," "I want to be toned." What tends to come out after a conversation are goals like, "I want to be able to run around with my kid" or "I don't want to have to ask for a seat-belt extender or buy a second seat." The goal should always be to be healthy, but health isn't defined by size. The goal should be to feel good in our bodies. The goal should be to push ourselves. If we want to be able to do something, then we have to try and do it.

There has been a lot of interesting talk within the body positive community over the last few years. Some people say if you really love your body, why should you work out? It means you want to change something about yourself, so you couldn't possibly be body positive. I understand that notion, but this is once again an idea that society has put into our heads: that exercise and fitness have to be about weight loss. Working out and exercising don't have to mean that you want to lose weight. It can actually be about being and feeling healthy (figure 1.1). Health is a continuum.

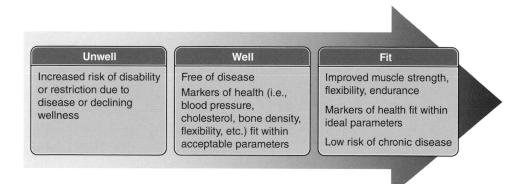

Figure 1.1   The health continuum.

When you go to the doctor, she takes basic measurements to assess where you generally fall on this continuum. Our blood pressure should be between 100/60 and 120/80, all within normal ranges. Our cholesterol should be under 200 mg/dL, and our resting heart rate should be between 50 and 100 bpm. The weight standards are there for a reason: Too much fat mass is detrimental to the systems of the body. However, what has been lacking in people's understanding is that weight doesn't always correlate to fat mass. A pound of feathers weighs the same as a pound of steel. The difference is density. I bring up these health standards to point out that our bodies' shapes and sizes should not be what stops us. We shouldn't be judged on what we look like. The fact that you weigh more than the person next to you doesn't mean that you are unhealthy. The size and shape of your body are not what matters. What matters is where the rest of your numbers are. But even then, it's not exactly the numbers that matter. Maybe you wake up every day and feel tired, or perhaps you aren't sleeping at night. Maybe your body aches or you have headaches or stomachaches all the time. It's not normal to feel sick every day. It is your body's way of telling you something. If we are eating well and sleeping and moving, we actually should have plenty of energy and should feel good.

WHEN THERE'S TOO MUCH (OR TOO LITTLE) INFORMATION

Instagram and social media have also changed the game in a lot of ways. We get to see what so many people are capable of, and we get to see the coolest things that people can do. Backflips, handstands, pull-ups—we want to do it as well. In some ways this is amazing—it is getting more people off the couch. Free information is widely available, and it has connected people who probably never would have been connected otherwise. In the plus-size world, it has given us the opportunity to shine, to show the world that we are just as beautiful and can be anything we want to be and do anything we want to do.

On the flip side, we see too much information all the time. There is a difference between motivation and inspiration, and that can get lost easily with the influx of information coming at us. We see that one expert says that all carbohydrates are bad, while another says that carbohydrates are good. One expert says don't let your knees pass your toes in a squat or lunge, and another says it's fine. (We will get to this one later.) We think *If I want to look like this person, I have to do everything she is doing.* I will tell you right now, she didn't tell you half of what she actually did—and by the way, you are not that person! We see a post with a transformation photo, someone who has lost a ton of weight or gained a ton of muscle. What isn't shown is all the hard work that went into it! What isn't shown is that in order to hit whatever goal you may have, there is a lot more happening than what is being shown in a couple of videos taken on a cell phone. And while it is important to feel a connection with someone,

I need to be clear that you shouldn't be buying workout programs from an Instagram model who works out. Please be sure to support the hardworking fitness professionals who have put in the time and effort in their field.

Look around you for a minute or think about your group of friends or family. Do you all have the same exact body? Do you all weigh the same and are you all good at only one thing? No! It doesn't work like that. I could eat the same exact thing as the person next to me and our bodies digest food differently. That's why some people can eat whatever they want and never gain any weight. You don't know what their insides are like. I can do the exact same training program as my friends—same weights, rest periods, reps, and sets; sleep the same number of hours; and drink the same amount of water in a day—and we still won't look the same. I don't think that is a bad thing. If anything, isn't it trendy to be unique? We can have similar goals. It is okay to want to lose weight or gain muscle mass, but you are still going to look like you and I'm still going to look like me. It's time to let go of the social norms and be happy with ourselves.

There are lots of forms of exercise, from running to dancing and Pilates to swimming. The most important thing is that we move. If you were to learn one lesson from this book, I would want it to be that movement is the most important thing. Yes, I'm biased toward strength training. I love it, and I hope to help you love it too, but the most important thing is to move. One of the reasons I love strength training so much is the purity of movement. Like I said before, there are fundamental movements that we all learn inherently. All forms of exercise come from the fundamental things our bodies are capable of. In order to be a dancer who can jump and leap beautifully, you need to be strong. In order to be a gymnast, you need to be strong. In order to carry your kids upstairs to bed, you need to be strong. I truly believe there is a place for all movement in fitness and exercise, and all movement requires some level of strength.

PRESSURE, PRESSURE, AND MORE PRESSURE

Pressure from the world, doctors, family, and friends to get healthy can be way too much for us to handle. Everyone has an opinion; everyone thinks you should lose weight, or wear this, or eat that. We should all have standing desks, only sleep on our backs, and own these sneakers that are the best for your knees. In a world filled with these pressures, we have to figure out what is best for us. What happens too often is you go to the gym because you feel you have to. I want to remind you to do this for you. If you don't want to do it, don't. No pressure. But if you want to try, let's do it!

Maybe your high expectations of the gym have left you disappointed. It's too hard, or you don't enjoy it. But instead of taking the time to find an activity that makes you happy, you don't go back. Or you continue to suffer through a fitness routine that you don't like. Why are you voluntarily doing something that you hate? Working out is voluntary, so if you do hate one kind of workout, try something else. If you hate lifting weights, it's okay. Try dancing, yoga, or swimming. Creating a habit of working out is hard, so make it easy on yourself. Be nice to your body, take some of the pressure off, and find something you like.

THE THINGS THAT MATTER

Habit, consistency, and enjoyment: These are all things that matter. Whatever your reasoning for starting a strength program, you need to create a habit—motivation and inspiration only get you so far. Habit is the key to consistency, which you also need. In order to get to the point of habit, I have to enjoy what I'm doing, at least a little bit. Let's take an example: I hate kale. I just don't like it. You and everyone else in the world could tell me how good kale is for me, that there are life-altering benefits, and I still won't enjoy kale. Maybe I should make myself eat it, but I definitely wouldn't enjoy it. So, I'd have it one day, but probably not the next. I won't be able to create the habit if I have to fight through the taste every time I try to eat it. Spinach, on the other hand, I love! So I eat my greens, but not the way you do.

When it comes to movement and exercise, for years I tried to like running. I have always been told that running is good for me. It's the best and fastest way to lose weight. Since elementary school, we are told we have to run (remember that presidential fitness test?). The pressures didn't stop after that. I work in a gym setting. It seems like running comes so easily to everyone else, but after running for only a minute, everything in my body would hurt and I couldn't breathe. I kept trying, and yes there were times in my life that I have been able to push through and run a few miles without stopping. But I still never enjoyed it. When something hurt, I would stop and once again feel defeated. I was never able to make it a habit. Why would I voluntarily do something that I don't enjoy? Lifting weights, on the other hand, I would do every day, all day, twice a day if I could. I love it. I can work hard, without pain. I'm good at it, and I'm not in a race with the guy lifting next to me. I'm not the slowest one on the track. We all have to find the thing that keeps us coming back. We have to do it for ourselves and no one else.

It's a funny thing I'm about to say, but it's the truth. I'm a personal trainer, a strength coach, and a fitness influencer, and yet I can't convince you to work out. I can do my best to motivate you, and I can do my best to check on you and make sure you are holding yourself accountable, but I can't do the work for you. I can make the work a bit easier: I can tell you exactly what to do, when to do it, and how to do it. But I can't do it for you. That's my next endeavor, being able to work out for people and they get the gains. (Okay, just kidding.)

Strength training teaches mental toughness. No one ever said exercise was easy. If you want to get stronger, you have to realize that there is going to be hard work involved. When we think we can't do another rep, we try anyway. When we think we can't hold that plank any longer, we hold for 10 more seconds. Strength training not only works to make you physically stronger but also to make you mentally stronger, too. You may have heard that "We all have stress in our lives; it's how you handle it." Well, that's true here, as well. Getting stronger takes dedication, which means you are a dedicated person. It means that you respect yourself. If you say you are going to do something and do it, that is self-respect. If we can push through physical discomfort, if we can push to do one more rep, if we can add a little weight to the bar, we can get through so much more. Being physically strong can also give you a new type of confidence. Confidence is something most people—in some way, shape, or form—lack. It's normal, but a lack of confidence can be detrimental to our overall health. Strength training can show you what you are made of, what you are capable of. From one week to the next, you can see physical strength improve. Seeing that improvement can help you stay on track; it can help you realize the hard work is paying off. I would never promote strength training as a quick and easy fix, but the truth is that you can and do see improvements all the time. No matter if you are a beginning, intermediate, or advanced lifter, you can see progress, both physically and mentally.

To get positive effects from building strength, we have to find the motivation within ourselves. Trying isn't as good as doing. I can tell you from personal experience that strength training—and working out, in general—has had so many benefits for me. I could list the benefits stated by doctors and research all day long, but would that motivate you to try it out? Strength training and working out is a part of who I am at this point. I'm single and I get asked on dating apps all the time: What are your hobbies, what do you like to do for fun? Work out, lift, play: Fitness is my life. I'm not expecting it to be your life; that's an unrealistic expectation. However, if you want to see and feel some of the benefits of lifting weights, you do have to make it part of your regular routine; it can't be a once-in-a-while activity.

A major benefit of fitness is learning discipline. Discipline usually isn't what people think of as a benefit, but we are creatures of habit. We thrive off of routine. Routine, whether we like it or not, is the best thing for us. Wake up, use the bathroom (don't forget that daily squat), brush teeth, wash face, put on clothes, eat breakfast, head to work, head to the gym, head home, eat dinner, go to sleep, and repeat. Your routine may look different, but it's still structure. Where does the discipline come in? Your alarm goes off, but you don't have to get up. You do it because you have to get to work on time. You do it because it's what you do every day, you don't think about it. You can have fun within the parameters of having discipline, but it can help us reach our goals.

THE STYLES OF STRENGTH TRAINING

Let's take a look at styles of strength training. There is bodybuilding, otherwise known as hypertrophy, which is muscle building and growth. There's powerlifting, which is true strength. You've got Olympic weightlifting, which is lifting really heavy weights with a lot of speed and control. And then there is total-body circuit training, which is best for the general population. It can be incredibly overwhelming. What works best for one person may not work for the next. What you should keep in mind is that if you are a beginner, it is best to start slowly and with some guidance.

Yes, I'm a personal trainer and a strength coach, and I'm writing a book about strength training because I love it and truly believe you will benefit from it. However, I honestly don't care what you do to move, as long as you move. As long as you start to move your body, you will start to see progress. You don't need a plan for that. As a beginner, changes happen rather fast; you see the most dramatic changes in the first six weeks of a strength program. To quote myself, "I don't care what you do, as long as you do something." I have worked with many new-to-fitness individuals. If you have been leading a sedentary lifestyle, adding any kind of movement is going to make a difference. If you have been a runner your whole life and you suddenly start lifting weights, you are going to see a difference. But finding the type of exercise that keeps you coming back is important. The point is, you have to start somewhere.

Generally, when you are looking to get stronger, the barbell is involved. Plenty of people disagree with me, but I've been doing this a long time, and I have worked with a lot of bodies. Dumbbells only go so high in weight, and the barbell allows you to add weight. Some individuals in the fitness industry I respect, but don't agree with, believe that anyone can start a fitness routine by picking up the barbell right away. I love the barbell; it's one of my best friends and I respect it. However, I believe that you have to master bodyweight movements first. I want people to strive to use a barbell. However, I also want you to take your time getting there.

THE IMPORTANCE OF REPRESENTATION

I mentioned before that growing up, I was only concerned about myself and how fat I was. I couldn't tell you if any other kids at school were fat, or if anyone else around me was fat. Within the last few years, with the rise of social media, we have all been stepping into the limelight. We are seeing people of all shapes, sizes, and colors everywhere. Unless you have been living under a rock, we are seeing more women of all shapes and sizes on TV and in advertisements. More clothing companies are making plus-size clothing. It opened my eyes in an interesting way and I realized that I wasn't alone.

But I also realized that there wasn't anything wrong with me. I started to notice that there were people in my life, and not just on social platforms, that were people of size as well. I know it sounds crazy, and probably a little selfish, but, really, no one has ever been fat in my eyes because I was only worried about myself. Roughly 67 percent of women are plus size in America. Clearly, it's not just me; once I freed myself of thinking I was alone, I was able to associate myself with people who not only are awesome but also get me. I've shared some of my story in the preface (page xi) about how and why strength training has become such a big part of my life.

Throughout this book, you will read stories of some amazing, strong women who have stories and journeys that I find inspiring, and I hope you do, as well. I hope that their stories will help us all remember that we aren't alone. I want these stories to remind you that you are not alone, and that we all have to start somewhere. The clear message across the board is that when you set your mind to do something, you can. When you decide that you are ready to make a change, the change happens. Each of these women speaks to how strength training has made them physically and mentally stronger. These are stories from women who weren't child athletes, who hadn't been working out their whole lives, but who made a decision that was totally scary and decided to try something new and to see what they were all capable of. These women lead very different lifestyles. I know them all personally. They are of all ages and in different stages of life. My point: You can start at any time and you will never know if you can succeed unless you try.

CONCLUSION

Take a moment and remember why you picked up this book in the first place. We all have our reasons for wanting to start on a fitness journey. I hope that whatever your reason, it is for you. I hope that you can put into practice being kind to yourself, patient, and ready to work hard. Please remember that there is a lot of information to help you be successful in this journey. If we were working one-on-one together, I would only give you one or two pieces of the puzzle at a time. I don't want you to feel overwhelmed about the amount of information that is out in the world or in this book. Take your time, read, and reread if needed. Start slowly, and practice self-love and patience.

PREPARE TO MOVE

Whether you want to start strength training for physical strength, mental strength, or general health, you are making the decision to change something about yourself that maybe you didn't like before. What is going through your mind that makes you want to make a change? "I'm so weak" or "I can't even do a push-up." In this chapter, you'll learn how to turn those negative thoughts into positive ones and the steps to make improvements that you can feel good about. And if you aren't having negative thoughts, you are already ahead of the game. Either way, what we talk about in terms of mindset will help you on this journey.

THE IMPORTANCE OF MINDSET

Mindset is probably the most important part of becoming strong. I can teach you how to squat and deadlift; that's easy. I can't make you want to work out. I can't make you want to be stronger. I can certainly help guide you, but you have to decide you want it on your own. You are the one who has to put in the work, and when the workouts are hard, you are the one who can decide to push through it and not give up. This is why taking the time to prepare yourself and change your mindset is essential. We have to commit.

We can do anything we set our minds to. But how do we actually start? You would think the first step is to start moving, and while that is important, the first step is making a change to your mental state. We must go into this with the right mindset. Take the time to decide that you truly want something and commit to it. This doesn't mean that you have to jump all in. It doesn't mean that we should make every change at once. It means that you have to commit to wanting change, that you will dedicate yourself to even the smallest of changes. In lifting, we talk about walking up to the bar with confidence. Well, if the first step is to walk into the gym, whether outside your house or in your own living room, walk in with confidence. Have you heard of superhero pose (figure 2.1)? Stand with your feet hip-distance apart, hands on your hips, and your chest up tall. In this pose, you are creating the impression that you are ready.

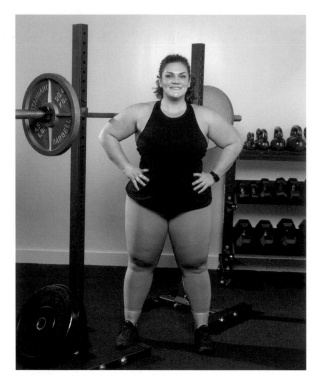

Figure 2.1   Superhero pose.

Find a mantra—a saying—and repeat it to yourself as you are taking that first step. When I am facing a new challenge, I make a plan ahead of time. For example, when I did my first Whole30 nutrition plan, I set a date that I was going to start it. I did some research; I prepared my mind and my kitchen. When I woke up on day one, I sat up in bed and said to myself, "Okay, Whole30, let's f-ing go!" I bring up that experience because initially when I was asked to do the Whole30 program with a group of people, I flat out said *no*. I didn't think I could do it; I didn't think I could give up chocolate for 30 days. I took some time to think about it and changed my mind. The biggest lesson I learned was that I could do anything I set my mind to. I also have a mantra for myself when I question why I do anything that's hard or challenges me. I say, "I want to be my best self." It's open-ended, but no matter the mental state I'm in, it pushes me to keep going. You might tell yourself, "I will be able to do X push-ups" or "I am strong." In my work, I hear the statement "I can't" way too often. If you have already decided you can't, you might as well go home. Materialize your goals into existence. Your goals and what's important in your life will change over time, and creating a positive mindset helps you get through it. No matter what your mantra is, only put good vibes out into the universe.

Can you come up with something right now? Wanting change is usually something we have been thinking about for a while, so there are probably already thoughts in your head that you can use as your mantra. Write it down.

Go ahead, write it down—right here. Write down a couple things. You can make changes later to your statements; nothing is set in stone. Goals or mantras I've had in the past have evolved and changed over time.

_____

_____

_____

_____

_____

_____

BODIES AREN'T ALL CREATED THE SAME

You have probably seen the videos on social media of people doing exercises wrong and people making fun of them. I have been in the gym and seen some really crazy stuff. Sometimes it is funny, but it's not okay to make fun of what people are doing. We need to do a better job of making people feel comfortable and keeping an open mind. Consider that people might not know any better, or there may be a reason someone is doing something differently. As a trainer, it's my job to help people who need it. It's my job to teach the movements to the best of my ability, but mainly to ensure safety.

Personal trainers teach proper form for each movement based on the way the body is built and works. There is a right way, and there are some not-so-right ways to do exercises. The only time something is completely wrong is if you are in danger. Many trainers don't take into account that different bodies move differently. We are all built differently; my hips may move differently than yours. For plus-size women, some movements need to be adjusted. For example, trainers use general cues to teach a squat. I usually ask a client to just squat. I don't give any cues at first, and then I wait to see what the person does. Sometimes it's perfect, and we don't need to fix anything. Other times, there's a simple fix. It takes time for the client to adjust technique so that it's effective and doesn't cause an eventual injury. However, if we break it down, these are the steps: I want you to sit and stand back up, arms straight out in front of you, feet turned out at about 30 degrees and about hip-width apart. Drive your hips back to the wall behind you. As you lower your body, drive your knees out to the sides and sit back until you find the chair. Stand back up. Once you are comfortable with this, you progress. Instead of sitting down, maybe you just tap the chair, and then hover over the chair. Eventually you are squatting.

Meet Anise

"To the fat women (and all people who have internalized the message that your body is wrong), I was a 10-pound baby. I've been fat since day one. I don't remember when I first internalized the message that my body was wrong, and that because I was, physical achievement would never be within my grasp. In grade school, then junior high and high school, I struggled through laps and presidential fitness tests, humiliated and alienated. The slow one. The sweaty one. I learned how to change in a room full of other girls without ever completely removing my clothes. Is this scene familiar? I often wonder what my relationship to my body and to health and fitness could have been if I knew then what I know now.

Though the resulting changes have been multifaceted, I started powerlifting for political reasons. I believe that physical strength is an avenue to accessing power. The ruling class holds power and thus, it is generally owned and safeguarded by men, especially straight white cis men. Strength is sequestered to those traditionally associated with physical ability, aggression, masculinity—power. Those of us who don't fit this description—fat people, women, trans, and queer people—are made to feel that strength is not for us and the spaces in which it is learned are built to exclude us. Accessing that power as a fat, queer, femme person of color is a political act. Women and femmes are told from birth that we are, first and foremost, ornamental. We must be docile, fragile, and beautiful. These characteristics are conflated with femininity and womanhood itself. We are told that we must be sexy while also virginal, nurturing yet vulnerable, and above all, beautiful. And to be beautiful, we must be small. Refusing to shrink is a political act.

I didn't understand all this as clearly as I do now. I did know that I wanted to feel less afraid and more capable. More than that, I wanted to be able to look in a mirror, not at my size or my shape, but at my life, and be proud of the person I was becoming. And yet gyms and fitness culture, as well as the theater and dance world in which I was deeply involved, only ever demanded thinness.

The first time I walked into CrossFit South Brooklyn in January 2016, I had never set foot in a box gym. I felt awkward and out of place. I flashed back to that high school locker room. Gyms can be scary places for fat people, especially femmes. I had been told all my life that I did not belong there, and that I was self-destructive, lazy, and stupid if I did not show up.

But a friend had loaned me a book called Starting Strength and explained how strength training might be different and really helpful for me. I walked in under the fluttering rainbow flags and met people who wanted not to help me be small, but to help me get stronger. I did my first workout and I felt like a superhero. Strength training was the first sport or physical arena in which no one was telling me that my body had to shrink in order to perform. Rather, the fact that I have a large body, a body with the genetic predisposition to grow, was not a hindrance but an advantage. I didn't know what it could be like to care for my body, to do something to help my body be healthier and more capable of getting through life without weight loss being the goal. What I looked like didn't matter. The focus was not on the ways in which my body falls short of some societal standard, but on how amazing my body is, how much it can do, and how to do more than the day before.

I had never and have never since experienced anything like the first time I added weight to the bar and squatted it successfully. The first time I lifted 135 pounds, 225, 315, my first total, my first meet. I felt pride, accomplishment, an unprecedented connection to my body, but above all—power. The results were immediate. Not the changes to my appearance (those have occurred very slowly and minimally over the last three years) but the changes to how my body feels, what I can physically accomplish, my approach to fitness and fitness environments, and how I carry myself through the world. Accessing that physical strength was transformative in that it opened the door to all the other ways in which I can empower myself and others. Powerlifting is walking up to a bar every workout, whether you are scared or not, whether you believe you can do it or not, and trying. It is failing and then coming back for the next workout. It has taught me self-discipline, courage, and dedication. Above all, it has taught me that strength and power can be achieved by anyone who is willing to fight for them."

Anise

I don't know about you, but this story gave me all the feels. I know Anise personally; we actually joke around in the gym all the time about who can lift more weight. I love it! I thrive off competition, but it's the friendliest competition you have ever seen. We truly and wholeheartedly only want each other to succeed. I watch Anise show up to strength class every week, ready to work. I've seen her compete with a smile on her face, and I've had the pleasure of having her cheer me on as well. What an honor it's been to be around such a confident, hardworking woman who also loves to lift heavy. What Anise did not mention in her story is that she is currently working on becoming a strength coach as well.

The way to tell if you are doing something right is if you are in pain or not. If it's painful, then your squat needs to be adjusted in some way. Keep in mind that there is a huge difference between discomfort that comes from working hard and pain. When you are new to movement and exercise, sometimes it's hard to differentiate between these feelings. The good news is that with time, you will learn the difference. If you squat and feel pain, it's wrong. You could be squatting exactly the way you were taught, but if it's painful, it doesn't work for you. Maybe you need to reposition your feet, either wider or narrower. Maybe you can squat to full depth but it hurts your knees when you do. Just because you were told to do it in a certain way does not make it right. If it hurts, it isn't right. As a plus-size woman, you may need to make adjustments so you can move in ways that work best for you. It might take a few tries to find the right way to do the movement for you. Your exercise might not look exactly like the next person, but that doesn't matter because all bodies aren't created the same.

That being said, in some situations there is a right way to perform a movement. For example, if you compete in lifting competitions, you have to meet specific standards. In order to get green lights on a squat, you have to hit a certain depth. If hitting depth is currently something that is hard for you, it doesn't mean that it always will be. It took me years to be able to sit into a full squat comfortably. I still spend a lot of time sitting in the bottom of a squat, breathing and letting my body know that I'm safe in this position.

In the upcoming chapters, I explain each of the movements that I feel are best for strengthening your body. I'll give basic cues to help you identify the best version of each movement for you. You may be surprised by what your body can do. You may not get it right away, and that's normal. Remember to be patient—this is a journey and a learning process.

GETTING STARTED

Step one, walking into the gym, is often harder than the workout itself! Remember this is a mental game. The workout itself isn't the hard part. Getting there, doing it, being willing to be uncomfortable; that's the hard part. The stress we put on ourselves, the blocks that we create—all of these are what make working out so difficult. If we think of a workout as something we get to do, versus something we have to do, the first step might immediately feel a bit easier. "I get to move today, I get to work out today, I get to feel strong today." Try some of these statements when you find yourself fighting step one. Because really, step one is the act of starting.

SETTING GOALS!

Let's start with how to set a goal. Your goal needs to be specific. What is it that you want to accomplish? While it's great to say, "I want to get stronger," what does that mean? There needs to be more to that statement. We want to be able to track progress; we want to be able to see improvement. Your goal on day one can be to get stronger. I talk to my clients about this all the time, that it's okay to get started in a general direction and then make more specific decisions along the way. The goal is to work to be healthier—and maybe your goal is just to feel good in your body and you don't care about seeing specific improvements. This works for some. However, one of the main reasons we set goals is to strive to improve. It's to get excited about seeing progress because this keeps us from stopping. Let's say your goal was to do 10 push-ups, and you worked from 0 to 8 push-ups in a couple months. Would you stop? Would you give up on your goals, on all the hard work you put in? Probably not. That goal gives you something to work toward.

Setting goals is all about the journey. It's important to know that it won't happen overnight. Recognize that putting in the work and seeing it come to fruition keeps you motivated. So, I encourage you to set a specific goal. Your goal should have a specific time frame in which you want to achieve it, and it also needs to be realistic. For example, "I want to squat 300 pounds, even though I have never barbell squatted before." What an amazing goal, one that will take a significant amount of time, especially if you are being safe and smart.

There are a couple things to keep in mind when setting goals. One is to create smaller goals along the way. In the barbell squat example, you might start with hitting 100 pounds, then 150, and so on. Second, you have to do a little math to figure out a realistic time frame. Generally speaking, if you follow a linear progression–style program (meaning you keep adding weight incrementally until you can't add any more), you should be able to add 5 to 10 pounds to your squat each week. This is a general statement, not exact. But if we were to make an estimate, in learning to squat the barbell, adding 5 to 10 pounds per week on top of the 45-pound barbell would take 5 to 12 weeks or more to get to 100 pounds. Linear progression programs for beginners work well because it's a start forward, and you see the most strength gains in the beginning.

But just to keep us all humble, we can't progress on a linear progression program forever because if we all could add 5 or 10 pounds per week to our squat from now on, I'd be squatting well over 1,000 pounds by now. When setting a time frame for your goals, remember that there will be bumps in the road and sometimes the time frame has to be adjusted. You should write down your goals and share them with important people in your life. Telling someone else what you plan to achieve makes it more real. Keeping it inside or a secret means you have no one to be accountable to. You should only be setting goals for you, but having the support of family and friends can make the difference in whether you achieve your goal or not.

Keep in mind, too, that you need to think about the sacrifices you are willing to make to achieve your goal, and your goal must be a priority. Nothing happens overnight. It takes hard work and effort. If I want to train hard in the gym, I may have to sacrifice staying out late with friends the night before. Or I may have to wake up at 6 a.m. to make sure I get my workout in before work. There are no excuses, just work-arounds. You have to make your goal the priority.

Last, you must develop a plan to achieve your goal.

Make a Plan

If you have considered your goals and decided on a workout plan to meet those goals (see chapter 6), it can keep you from feeling lost and getting injured. It can help keep you on track because you have a purpose for your workouts besides just "needing to work out."

Once you have determined what you are going to do and how, it's time to get to the movement. What comes along with the movement and the exercises is also important to understand. Any time someone starts a new workout program, the body is going to feel different—maybe a little beat-up and sore. This is why a plan of action is so important; if we go in on day one and do too much exercise, our bodies have a hard time recovering. Starting slowly is key. The body can handle only so much, especially at first. Sore is okay, and stiff is okay. Unable to walk at all? You probably overdid it.

Progress can be slow as you start lifting, and knowing when to make yourself work harder can be tricky. You might want to do the challenging variation or to add more weight. But is it appropriate? Before you make a lift more difficult, ask yourself a few questions:

- Do I feel safe?
- Do I trust myself with this movement?
- Can I perform this movement without thinking too much?

We all want to be able to lift more weight or do the higher box jump, but it takes time. Be patient with yourself!

Schedule Your Workouts

Now that you have a goal in mind, make time in your life to devote yourself to this new priority. You may wonder, "How often should I go to the gym?" Movement can happen seven days a week, and we should be moving our bodies. However, when it comes to lifting weights, the body needs rest. Rest days are needed to let your body recover, and they are also great to use as planning and prepping days.

Figuring out the answer to how many days a week you work out depends on a few things: What is your goal? How often is it practical for you to work out? Are you a beginner, or have you been doing this a while? For beginners, the first thing I ask is, "What is reasonable and realistic?" If clients tell me they can work out four or five times a week, I often prescribe three or four.

Remember when I talked about consistency in chapter 1? It doesn't matter if you *can* go four or five times per week; it matters that you actually go. Lifting weights three or four times a week is fantastic, whether a beginner or experienced lifter. When you are on a strength training program, there are different ways to split it up. If you have three or four days available, you would be doing full-body workouts each of those days. When lifting five days a week, the program might split into lower-body and upper-body days. Many of my clients lift two times per week with me because that's how many personal training sessions they can afford, then they do a third day on their own. These workouts can involve lifting weights or cardio. It depends on their goals.

For a beginner, doing anything new is going to make a huge difference. I have worked with new clients who found that lifting twice a week made them stronger. There are 168 hours in a week. I ask that you dedicate at least three of those hours to lifting. Remember that you must move every day, even if that's walking half a mile at first. You won't see much change if you only do intentional movement once a week.

And here's something else to consider when deciding how often you want to lift weights. Lifting doesn't have to be the only thing. Our goals determine whether we specialize in one activity or enjoy a variety of ways to move our bodies. If your goal is to be the strongest person in the world, then you probably need to lift exclusively and not also go to spin class. If your goal is to be strong and healthy, lifting and spin class can go hand in hand. Lifting places more load and strain on the body than a spin class, so lifting should be your first priority. Lifting weights can be very taxing, so it is a good idea to lift first and then move on to cardio. This is not a must. Try both ways and see how you feel and perform during your workouts. If you start with cardio and go to lift and have no energy left, ask yourself if that made the most sense for you, and vice versa.

Look at the week ahead and schedule your workout time like you would any other appointment. My calendar is shared in figure 2.2 as an example.

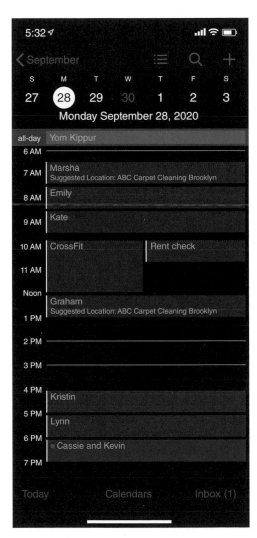

Figure 2.2   Sample workout calendar.

Choose Your Workout Clothes

Lay out your gym clothes the night before your workout. Make sure you are wearing something that makes you feel comfortable and confident. Hooray for plus-size fashion. For years, I would wear oversized sweatpants and sweatshirts when I worked out. I was constantly adjusting my clothes and didn't want to do certain exercises because I knew my clothing would be a distraction. I was always worried about my pants falling down or my stomach jiggling. I wore two bras—a regular underwire bra and a sports bra on top—to make sure that I wouldn't have a bouncy situation. I was already uncomfortable in my skin, and the clothing situation didn't make it any better.

I remember buying my first pair of leggings that actually fit. My whole world changed. My entire attitude changed. I remember finally finding sports bras that fit and tops that were comfortable. Luckily, now that the world of fashion for plus-size women has changed, there are brands that make workout apparel for different body sizes. There are major brands that go up to 5x, which was not the case when I started in the fitness industry. I highly recommend finding clothing that you don't have to constantly adjust and a pair of pants that passes the squat test. Find a bra that you are comfortable in that doesn't let the girls fly free. A good pair of leggings has just the right amount of compression and won't slide down. Many of these brands are affordable, but make sure they are good quality. You are investing in yourself. There is nothing more distracting than a pair of leggings you have to adjust while you are lifting. Our attention shouldn't be on anything other than the workout. Some brands have styles they recommend for specific workouts. I say find what you feel comfortable in. You can find brands with great return policies now, so try stuff out and see how you feel. Once I find something I like, I own it in every color.

NUTRITION BASICS

Let's talk about basic nutrition for recovery purposes. I want to remind you that making too many changes at once is not conducive to success. I'm not here to tell you I know everything about nutrition, and I'm not a registered dietitian, so I definitely won't tell you exactly what you should be eating.

Water

Water! Water! And more water! If you don't already do so, you should be drinking plenty of water. Our bodies can't function without water. More than half of our body weight is made up of water. But we lose water throughout the day by sweating, using the bathroom, even breathing.

There are plenty of ways to calculate or estimate the amount of water we should be drinking throughout the day, but the best calculator is your body. If you are thirsty, you have probably already hit levels of dehydration. Be sure to

Meet Maria

"My name is Maria DeMesa, and I'm a competitive powerlifter. I currently hold the drug-tested California state record for raw (with knee sleeves) squats at 420 pounds. I started in October of 2018 and haven't looked back. Before powerlifting, I was into competitive kettlebell sport for about two to three years. The communities for both strength sports are so empowering, and I have met so many amazing people.

Before strength sports, I played soccer from the age of 8 to 28. While I loved the sport, there was an aspect of feeling like my body didn't belong, that I was always going to be the biggest body on the field, and that it was a problem unless I was used as a goalkeeper. It obviously wasn't a problem, but I was surrounded by mostly visibly smaller people. Growing up, I was always one of the biggest bodies in my classrooms, and I stood out. I was made fun of and my self-esteem was never high enough to either not care or not think all of the hurtful things said to me were true. That was true up until I was 25 and pregnant with my now 8-year-old daughter.

Shortly before finding out I was pregnant, I was diagnosed with fibromyalgia. My mom, grandma, and two of my aunts also had it, so I was familiar with it. It completely shattered the world I once knew but put into perspective some of the weird pains I had had over the years. For most of my adulthood up until that point, I was made to believe that my large body was the problem. That I just needed to lose weight to feel better. So it was nice to finally have an answer, but it also meant I needed to rethink how I would move around in the world from that point forward. Two months after my diagnosis I found out I was pregnant.

I found strength sports in 2013 at a gym in Huntington Beach, California. Before that, I refused to touch a barbell because I bought into the ideas that "muscles equals bad" and that any type of weightlifting would make me bulky. Once I joined this gym, I was surrounded by all types of bodies. Due to it being a small, private class–based gym, I got to know people rather quickly, and everyone was so welcoming. That type of environment pushed me out of my exercise comfort zone, and it didn't take long for me to sign up for their strength sport classes.

Strength sports made me feel unlike I had ever felt before. It was empowering to know how naturally strong I was. It let me reframe how I thought about my larger body. I actually enjoyed every minute of it. This was new to me.

Fast forward to today, I love my larger body. My daughter is growing up with a mother who is not only physically strong but also has better mental and emotional health. Strength sports have taught me to love myself and let myself take up as much space as I need to without trying to shrink my body to fit society's mold of what a "healthy female"

(continued)

Meet Maria *(continued)*

should look like. That same mindset is now being passed down to my daughter and also up to my mother.

While society still has some unlearning to do, strength sports provide me a safe place to feel like I belong and that I have value."

Maria

For some people, strength training leads to competition, which is awesome. Powerlifting competitions are an amazing experience because you get to go out there and test yourself. These competitions aren't just a test of how much you can lift, but also a true test of your mental strength. It takes a lot to get up in front of a crowd and perform. A lot of energy goes into walking up to a platform, remembering everything you were taught, and giving the lift everything you've got. I'm not saying you should sign up for a meet right now. Training for a meet can be a great goal to ensure that you make it to the gym. I have worked with many lifters, and the one thing I tell them all is that we have to respect the process. If you want to lift in a meet, you have to train for it. It doesn't matter if you are lifting the most or the least, it matters that you worked just as hard as the next person to be there. In truth, many of us won't ever win first place—so it can't be about the win; it's about so much more. I bring up competing because it is probably one of the very few times that you would only focus on the activity at hand.

listen to what your body is telling you. I don't go anywhere without my water bottle. I like water, so it's easy for me to drink. If you have a hard time drinking water, ask yourself if you like warm or cold water. Don't listen to those who say cold water is bad for you or warm water won't burn any calories. It's water! I love cold water, so I carry a bottle that keeps my water cold. You can add natural flavors to your water such as lemon or cucumber. Find something that works for you. Take small sips throughout the day.

Food

Start slowly with the changes you make. Maybe the only change you make for the first two weeks is to consume more water. Once you have adapted to consuming the added water, maybe the next thing you do is focus on your vegetable intake.

If I were to give you some basic rules on food, they would be to eat food given to us from the earth: vegetables, fruit, meat, fish, and poultry. Whole food is natural. If your food comes in a package and has a long shelf life, it's probably manufactured and processed. The easiest way to make changes to your diet is to start here. Eat more foods that come from the earth and are not created by people. I mentioned vegetables first because they have high nutritional value but are also mostly water. Make sure you are eating a handful of vegetables at every meal. This can help hydrate you, keep you full longer, and keep you healthy overall.

I'm not going to go too deep into nutrition, but understand that no matter how hard your workouts are, if you aren't fueling your body properly, it is much harder to see results. And I'm not talking about weight loss, I'm talking about performance. So many times, when food gets mentioned, people immediately think we are going to talk about diet. Calories are like gasoline for a car. The car can't drive if it runs out of gasoline, and a body can't function without calories. Fueling the body—and understanding the purpose of fuel—is important if you want to be able to lift a lot of weight.

We have to fuel our bodies to function. People want to know if they should work out on an empty stomach. There is no absolute answer for this question because it depends on what you are doing and who you are. If you plan on lifting heavy, doing a strength-based workout, then it's a definite no. If you are going to do some light cardio, then maybe you can get away without eating before your workout. If you are working out in the early morning, getting in a meal prior to a workout can be hard. It doesn't have to be a whole meal, maybe just a snack. It takes time to figure out what foods you can handle so close to a workout. Everyone's digestion is different, so what works for you might not work for the next person. But fuel is fuel, and we need it to perform at our best.

You may have heard that people who lift weights need to take in extra protein, typically consumed in the form of a powder. It's not a requirement to use protein powder when you start lifting weights. Protein powder can work as an effective supplement if you don't get enough protein in your diet, but it is unnecessary if you eat a well-rounded diet. The two major types of protein powder are whey and casein. Whey is a fast-digesting protein, so usually it is consumed before, during, or directly after workouts to help replenish and fuel the body. Casein is a slow-digesting protein usually ingested before bed to help replenish the body.

However, we should be trying to get our fuel from natural sources. When I first started lifting, everyone had a pretty shaker bottle with their protein powder, so of course I ran straight to the store to get one, too. I used my shaker bottle and protein powder for a long time because I was convinced I wouldn't get stronger without it. How could I get through my workout without my protein? Then later, when I did the Whole30 nutrition plan for the first time, I couldn't use protein powders because they have tons of sugar in them. And you know what? I didn't feel a difference at all. Currently I don't take any supplements except for fish oil and a probiotic. I much prefer to eat a meal than to drink a protein shake. If you are eating protein throughout the day, there is no real need to jump on the protein powder train. However, if you are lifting heavy and not getting in enough protein, you may need to supplement.

STRENGTH TRAINING EQUIPMENT

Whether you want to work out from home or are going to the gym, there are only a few things that you need to get started.

Depending on what you can afford, resistance bands are a great tool. I could write a whole book about how to use resistance bands for strength. Many of the movements listed in chapters 3, 4, and 5 can be done with resistance bands. Depending on your goals, adding more load than you can get with a resistance band is necessary, but to start any fitness journey a resistance band can be helpful.

If you want to lift from home, kettlebells, dumbbells, and (depending on space and money) a squat rack, some plates, and a bench are all you need. For a beginner, I recommend a pair of lighter dumbbells (5-15 pounds), one or two heavier kettlebells, and a medium monster (long-loop) resistance band. You can make the weights heavier with the resistance band. If you find, as you progress, that you want to build up your home gym, get a squat rack or adjustable squat stand, a barbell, and some bumper or round plates to give you the ability to do all of the major strength lifts. Remember that a little can go a long way. Adding weight isn't the only way to work on strength, and we will be talking about that more in the upcoming chapters.

Finally, to help recovery, a foam roller is a great tool to have. Foam rolling the body not only feels good, but there are many stretches you can do to assist movements. I recommend getting a full-length (three feet), medium-density foam roller to start—no reason to get any of the fancy rollers at first. Learning how to foam roll isn't that hard. You can use books and online videos. It takes practice to get comfortable moving around on the roller. You should be rolling only on muscle, not joints. And if you can't breathe because it hurts too much, stop!

ACCESSORIES FOR STRENGTH TRAINING

Besides protein powder, there are so many accessories in the lifting world. I definitely won't be getting any sponsorships for saying this, but all you really need is your body. My body is the most important item I have. I don't need the newest sneakers, protein powder and a shaker bottle, or the newest gym bag; I need to show up and put in the hard work.

Even so, certain items can make workouts more efficient and maybe even more enjoyable. In strength training, you see lots of stuff: lifting shoes, weight belts, gloves, straps, wraps, chalk, and much more. Here, we'll look at some of these items so you can determine if they might be helpful to you.

Lifting Shoes

Lifting shoes are a great investment for someone who is dedicated to powerlifting and possibly competing. However, lifters (as they are sometimes labeled) do not make you lift more, they can't fix your squat, and they aren't required!

Lifters help with the positioning of the ankle at the bottom of the squat. Some people put weight plates under their feet to help them sit deeper into a squat. While there is a time and place for that, we don't want to mask ankle mobility issues. Without question, lifting shoes make it easier to squat deeper, but we shouldn't be completely dependent on using them. Lifters also cost a pretty penny; a good pair runs $150 and above. Instead of running out to get lifting shoes, let's do some ankle mobility work instead. I would recommend wearing a hard sole and flat shoe when lifting; too much cushion will prevent you from feeling the floor.

Weight Belts

Weight belts function to provide feedback about your technique. Breathing and creating tension are a huge part of lifting heavy weights. (We'll go into more detail later about how to breathe when lifting.) The weight belt is not required, nor is it something you should get on day one. In fact, it isn't something that should be used until you're ready for it. Using a belt too early can be detrimental to developing core strength.

Lifting Gloves, Wraps, Straps, and Chalk

Gloves: Leave them at home. Yes, your hands hurt for a little while after some lifts. But if you are wearing gloves you are blocking nerve endings in your hands from helping you get strong. Proprioception, which is another sense of the body like hearing and seeing, is awareness. We have to feel where we are in space. You need to feel to lift, and the way you need to feel is by using your hands. Proprioception can be lost with the use of gloves (or even shoes). We need to be able to feel the weights, feel the ground, and find our connection to the earth to create force. Lifting gloves come between you and the weight—and can dampen the signals from the nerve endings in your hands to the rest of the body that tell you to grip harder. Calluses take time to form, but they are the best kind of war wound, a badge of honor. Calluses do need a little care, and a simple emery board works. Filing down your calluses prevents tears in the skin. Grip strength is so important to work on, especially if the goal is to lift all the weights!

Speaking of grip strength, there are wraps and straps and so many other accessories. No need to rush to buy anything; build that grip strength without the aid of these tools until they are necessary. Wait until you are doing high-volume repetitions, holding the bar for a very long time, which may burn out your grip. Burnout simply means you can't hold on to the weight anymore. Feeling the burn in your muscles is something people think that they always need to strive for. That definitely isn't true. Burning muscles is normal and depending on what you are doing, you will feel it and you should push through some of it—let it burn. But when we lift heavier weights for a lot of reps—for example, a deadlift—our legs may still have the stamina to continue the movement but our grip strength gives out. This is an example of when a lifting strap would be appropriate. I'd suggest trying to lift without the straps for as long as you can; let your grip and forearms burn a bit.

Chalk is helpful if you have sweaty hands, but don't "over" chalk because it will lead to buildup and can cause your hands to slip. Use a small coating to prevent the weights from slipping.

All of these accessories for lifting can be great to have once you have been lifting for a long time but are unnecessary when you first start. If you are a beginner, you should be focused on form and technique for all your lifting. The weight is something that you will slowly increase. As I mentioned before, as a beginner you see pretty fast strength gains. Once you start to hit a plateau in your lifting, that will be a good time to consider if any of these accessories would help you. Accessories don't necessarily get you past your plateau, but sometimes they can help.

Mirrors and Cameras

You can use tools to help you figure out if your form is correct and safe. Mirrors and cameras can be helpful if you don't have access to a personal trainer or another person's eyes to see your movements.

I find that for certain things, mirrors are incredibly helpful because you sometimes need to see what you are doing. However, I prefer that you primarily learn to feel your body doing the movement. If your goal is to lift heavy, a mirror is not going to help you and could actually be unsafe. For example, if I'm deadlifting a weight that is heavy for me and I'm looking in the mirror, my neck is not in proper position. We will discuss proper alignment for deadlifts in later chapters, but when deadlifting you should be looking at the ground, so trying to look in the mirror can be unsafe to your cervical spine. For beginners, however, a glance in the mirror, before you actually lift the weight, to check if your back is rounded or if your arms are straight might be a helpful tool.

Cameras, which are found in most phones, are an accessible tool we can use to see what we're doing when we lift. You can set up your phone to record video or take photos of yourself doing a movement. This lets you look for consistency in your form or technique, to see what you might be able to improve. It takes time to learn what to look for, but using your camera helps you coach yourself.

And remember, just because you filmed yourself does not mean you are required to post it to Instagram!

Here are some tips for filming: You want to be able to see if you are hitting depth, if your back is flat, if your neck is in line, if you are hitting full range of motion on movements, and if your knees are buckling. Most of the time, filming from the side is the best angle. Take a squat, for example. I want to be able to see if I squat to depth, if my chest stays tight (up), if my lower back rounds. The thing you might miss from the side angle is if my knees buckle, so filming from the side but slightly in front is also a good idea. This slightly front side angle works with most movements.

STRENGTH TRAINING TERMINOLOGY

Become acquainted with these terms that you come across when lifting:

- **Rep**: A repetition is one complete and full range of motion of a single exercise. Repetitions are the number of times you repeat a movement within any given set.

- **Repetition max (RM)**: The number of times you can lift a weight. A 10RM is a weight you can theoretically lift 10 times and a 1RM is a weight you can lift one time. I say theoretically because these numbers are usually based on percentages of weight you have lifted in the recent past. We use these numbers to prevent overtraining and to estimate what you can lift.

- **Set**: A set is consecutive repetitions of a single exercise. Most programs are written as sets x reps, for example: 3 sets of 10 reps may look like 3x10.

- **Rest period**: A rest period is how long between sets you take to let your body recover before going back for more. Rest periods vary depending on your goals. In strength training, the goal is to lift a lot of weight. In order to recover, rest 1 to 5 minutes between sets, depending on how taxing the workout is. If you are doing a superset or a circuit, there will also be a rest period between exercises.

- **Superset**: Doing two exercises back-to-back with no rest other than to transition to the next movement.

- **Circuit**: Doing multiple exercises back-to-back with no rest other than to transition between movements.

- **Concentric**: The shortening of a muscle. For example, a concentric contraction during a biceps curl occurs when you bring the weight up. The concentric phase usually happens at the start of the movement.

- **Eccentric**: The lengthening of a muscle. In a biceps curl, the eccentric contraction occurs when you lower the weight. The eccentric phase usually happens when you are finishing the movement.

- **Push**: During push movements, you push a weight away from the body. A push movement could be a horizontal push (push-up) or a vertical push. (shoulder press). In these movements, I'm pushing weight away from my body.

- **Pull**: During pull movements, you pull a weight closer to the body. The deadlift is a vertical pull, and a row is a horizontal pull. I'm bringing weight closer to my body.

- **Hinge**: A hinge is a movement that means bending at the hips. In fitness, a hinge would also be a deadlift. It is usually described as bending downward and in half. I like to describe hinging as pushing my hips to an object behind me.

- **Compound movements**: In compound movements, exercises are combined to work more than one muscle group. A squat is a compound movement because it uses several sets of muscles in your body. Another example is a squat to press because you are doing two movements at once.

- **Isolation**: In an isolation exercise, you are focused solely on one muscle group. A biceps curl is a good example of an isolation exercise.

- **Isometric**: During an isometric exercise, you hold a movement in place. A plank is a great example of an isometric exercise.

- **Bilateral**: Bilateral means using both sides at the same time. If I do biceps curls with a weight in each hand and they move at the same time, this is bilateral.

- **Unilateral**: Using one side at a time. If I do biceps curls with a weight in each hand, but I lift only one weight at a time, this is unilateral.

- **Alternating (ALT)**: Changing sides. Let's use the biceps curl as an example. I could do a regular biceps curl, moving both of my arms at the same time (bilateral); perform a set using one arm at a time (unilateral); or I could perform an alternating biceps curl during which I switch arms at the end of each repetition.

- **Range of motion (ROM)**: Range of motion describes the degree through which each joint can work. Working through range of motion when lifting is important to keep our joints healthy and strong. When doing a biceps curl, I make sure that my elbow is fully lengthened before lifting the weight again. That is full range of motion.

- **Time under tension (TUT)**: The amount of time a muscle is under strain. During repetitions or while holding a position, you are under tension. This is where you might start to incorporate tempo training, slowing down and doing the movement with control.

- **Free weights**: Free weights are objects that provide load but are not attached to anything. You can move them freely in any capacity. Free weights are different from machines because machines determine your path of movement. When you use free weights, you determine the path of movement.

I've used machines many times, and they have their place. However, free weights are considered more functional. We train to live life. When we live life, we don't move in mechanical ways and we don't move with a perfect movement path, so using free weights simulates real-life movement better than machines do. You may see abbreviations used for common free weights, such as DB (dumbbell), BB (barbell), and KB (kettlebell).

CONCLUSION

It all starts from within—a positive attitude, a positive mindset, and a decision that you want to work hard for something. It starts by making the decision, coming up with a plan, and sticking with it. There are so many things within fitness to learn, but you do just have to start. You don't need anything but your body and your mind. Yes, learning movement is an important step, but it's not the hardest step. Try to block out all the noise when it comes to fitness—competing opinions and products and ways to hit your goals. I'm deep in the fitness industry, and I block out most of it. What most of the noise fails to mention is that in the end, movement is movement, and we are creatures made to move. If we let our natural instinct to move take over, most of the time that is the right direction. In the next few chapters, I teach the movements that are most important to help you start your strength training journey. Take your time, don't get frustrated, listen to your body, and remind yourself why you are here.

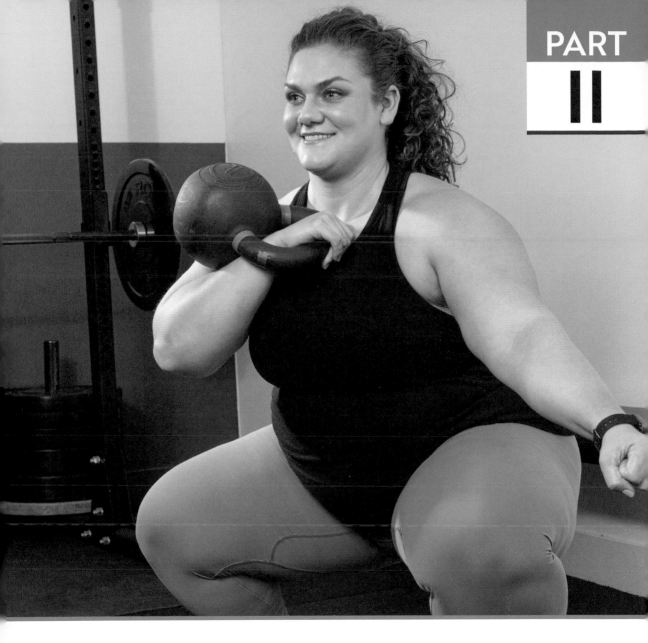

Get Moving

SQUAT AND HINGE

Let's dive in! This is the best part: learning each movement. In this chapter we are going to go through the squat and hinge patterns. The squat and hinge patterns form the basis for other exercises. They are also movements that you do in your everyday life. We will go through tips and tricks that help make these movements more efficient and safer when adding weight. Each exercise has variations; each variation changes the muscles used a bit—but, generally speaking, the main muscle groups stay the same. Do what works for you.

As plus-size women, we make adjustments for our bodies that vary from movement to movement. The main thing to keep in mind is to start slowly with a variation that works for you and gradually progress from there.

Squat and hinge movements mainly focus on the legs. The legs have muscles that you wouldn't even think about. Leg strength is necessary for everyday movement. From sitting down to standing up to walking up a flight of stairs, we need our legs to be strong and to function well. Each exercise featured in this chapter helps build strength that can be applied to everyday movement. A few major muscles are used in nearly every exercise, even if they aren't predominantly used. Muscles are still working.

The big muscle on the front of the leg that makes up the thigh is called the quadriceps. *Quad* means four. The four muscles that make up the quadriceps are used to extend the knee (straighten the leg) and to flex at the hip (sit down or bring the knee toward the chest). The hamstring makes up the back of the thigh. The three major hamstring muscles bend the knee and extend the hip (stand up). Last, but definitely not least, are the glute muscles—the butt! This is one of the most important muscle groups in the body. The glutes help us stand, sit, walk, run, and squat. The legs have other muscles (figure 3.1), but these three major muscle groups are the most important to understand when you are first getting started. For plus-size women who have large thighs and butts, the major thing to keep in mind is that position matters when doing exercises. Try different variations. You work the same muscles, but you may need to change your position to make the exercise work for you.

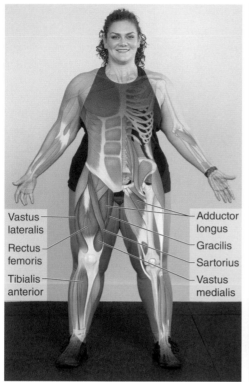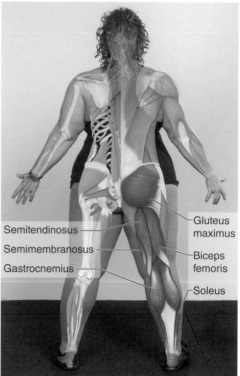

Figure 3.1   Muscles of the lower limbs.

Using a Squat Rack

Usually a squat rack requires only a few adjustments to make it work for you. Some squat racks have what are called *squat stands*; the two sides need to be put into place at a distance that works for you. The best distance usually is determined by the length of the barbell you are using. Any squat rack has *J-hooks* that hold the bar in place. Barbells have loading sleeves on both ends. The loading sleeves need to be outside of the J-hooks. Use this distance to help determine how wide to place your squat stand. No matter what kind of squat rack or stand you use, the most important aspect is where the J-hooks go. Usually you can determine the height of the J-hooks by standing next to one and putting it just below shoulder level. Test them with the bar first. If you have to go up on your tippy-toes to rack and unrack the bar, it's too high and should be lowered.

Squat

Sit down. It's just that simple. A squat is something you do every day; you sit down and stand back up again. That's step one. A squat is about learning to sit down and stand back up without using your arms to help you. It's about learning how to sit down with control.

Personally, the squat is my favorite movement. It took me a long time and a lot of practice to get good at the barbell back squat, but the process is why I love it so much. Not all pieces of the puzzle matter at first. Just being able to complete the movement is step one. Then we focus on efficiency; then adding weight, breathing, and proper bracing; and finally continuing to get stronger and respect the bar and your body.

Muscles

Primary: Gluteus maximus, quadriceps

Secondary: Hamstrings, erector spinae, adductors, calves, abdominals

Instructions

From a standing position, step the feet about hip-width apart with the toes turned out to about 30 degrees (figure 3.2a). You may find you need to have your feet wider or narrower, depending on your body. Find a position that allows a full-depth squat but in which you still feel comfortable. Think *belly strong*: Take a big inhale into your belly, hold your breath, and brace. Keep your chest up and your shoulders tight. Push your hips back and lower yourself toward the floor as you drive your knees out to the sides (figure 3.2b). Once your thighs are parallel to the floor, while maintaining tension, continue to drive the knees out to stand back up. Once you are at the top, you can exhale and repeat. That may seem like a lot of steps to squat, but it all happens rather quickly once you feel comfortable with it.

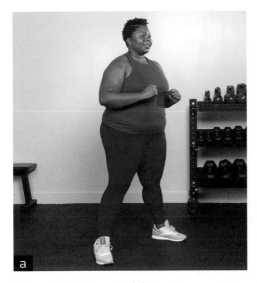
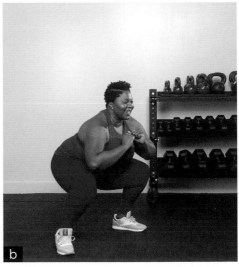

Figure 3.2 Squat: *(a)* starting position; *(b)* squat.

Movement Focus

A squat really is that simple, but there are factors that can get in the way of having the most efficient form. Trainers may see issues such as the knees buckling in, which can mean poor glute engagement. This is when the cue "drive your knees out" comes in handy. This cue reminds you to use your glutes as much as possible and prevent the knees from caving in. Trainers may also see clients not hitting depth if they start in positions that don't allow their bodies to move through a full range of motion. This problem can be caused by poor ankle, knee, or hip mobility, but fixing it is often as simple as standing a little wider and creating space to sink into your hips. Other inhibiting factors may stop people from hitting full depth, and that's okay. Sit to a depth that works for you. Some women never hit full depth; others just need practice and patience to get there. Last, fallen or collapsed chests during a squat can happen with or without additional weight. Remember when you are lifting, we want to create tension; keep good, strong posture, and use your whole body—core, back, and chest—to squat. When the whole body works together, it helps you keep your chest up and strong. If you were to sit with very poor posture right now and let your chest collapse all the way in and your back round, this would be the opposite of what we want when we are lifting.

Cues

- Breathe deep into the belly.
- Drive your hips back and your knees out.
- Set your feet hip-distance apart.
- Turn the toes out slightly.
- Hold your chest up.

Wall Test

To help you learn the feel of a squat, try the wall test. Stand about one foot in front of a wall, facing the wall. Place a low box or stability ball behind you. Get into your squat stance and place your hands behind or over your head. Your goal is to squat without falling backward or hitting your face on the wall. This test helps you feel your back muscles engage while squatting. Although the squat is a leg exercise, it involves the whole body.

Variations

Bodyweight Box Squat

Stand with a box or chair a few inches behind you (figure 3.3*a*). This box or chair should be at the height where you feel comfortable. You should be able to find the box with your butt with control and not fall; find a height that works for you. Set up in squat position. Sit your hips back and drive your knees out. Keep sitting back until your body finds the box (figure 3.3*b*). Depending on your needs, you can sit down or you can stay in the squat with tension and barely feel the box under your butt before standing up.

It may help with balance to hold your arms straight out in front of you and keep them strong. As you feel stronger, bring your arms closer and closer to the body. A box squat can be used for several reasons. Sometimes it helps to have a tactile cue to hit depth. Other times the box may calm a person's nerves. Often our heads are what get in the way. The box helps some of us get over our fear. In a worst-case scenario, you can sit down.

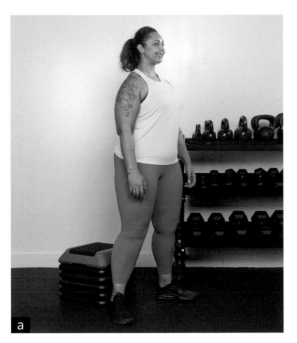
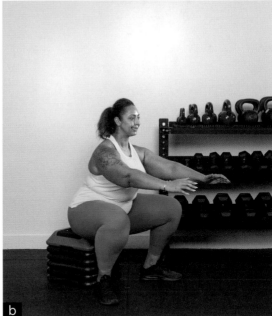

Figure 3.3 Bodyweight box squat: *(a)* starting position; *(b)* squat.

Prisoner Squat With Arm Variations

Follow the instructions for the squat movement: Stand with your feet hip-distance apart, toes turned out about 30 degrees, hips back, and knees out. To help keep your balance as you squat, place your arms out in front of you, either parallel to the floor or bent. To make your squat more challenging, place your hands behind your head with your elbows bent (figure 3.4) or reach straight overhead. Remember to keep your chest up, which is harder to do with the arms lifted.

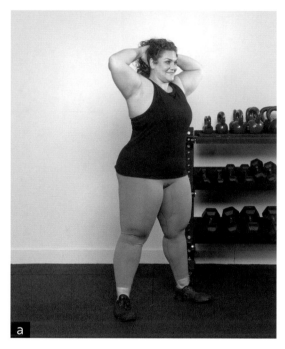 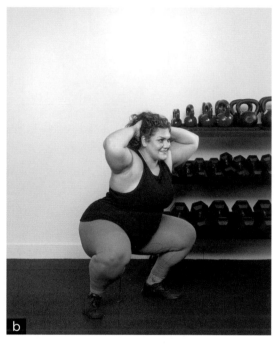

Figure 3.4 Prisoner squat with the hands behind the head and elbows bent: (*a*) starting position; (*b*) squat.

Goblet Squat

The same rules apply, but we now add a weight in front of the body. Hold any weight—a dumbbell, a medicine ball, or a kettlebell—at your chest (figure 3.5a). Stand with the feet hip-distance apart, toes turned out about 30 degrees. Drive your hips back and your knees out. As you squat, the weight tries to pull you forward. Now is the time to work to stay upright. Use your back to stay strong (figure 3.5b).

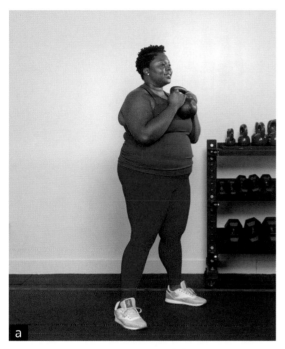 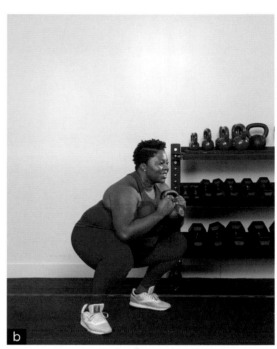

Figure 3.5 Goblet squat: (a) starting position; (b) squat.

Front Rack Squat

The front rack squat is usually done with two kettlebells. All the same rules of a squat apply, except you will place the kettlebell weight on the outside of the wrists (figure 3.6). Holding your weights at your chest, stand with the feet hip-distance apart and the toes turned out about 30 degrees. Drive your hips back and knees out. As you are sitting into your squat, focus on keeping your chest up so that the weight in your hands does not pull you forward. When heavy weight is put in front of the body, it tries to pull us down and forward. Hold your body upright and stay strong. Instead of kettlebells, dumbbells can be used with a slightly different setup (figure 3.7). A front rack squat with a barbell is called a front squat. It has a different setup with the bar but is the same concept. The weight is in front of you, and you build strength by working to keep your torso upright.

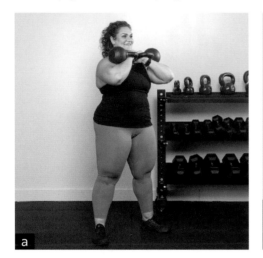
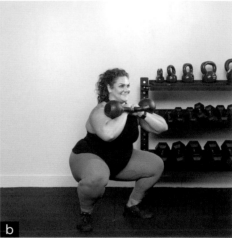

Figure 3.6 Front rack squat with two kettlebells: *(a)* starting position; *(b)* squat.

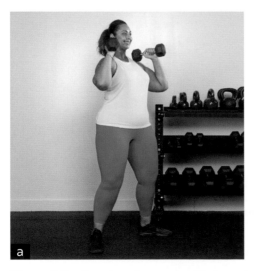
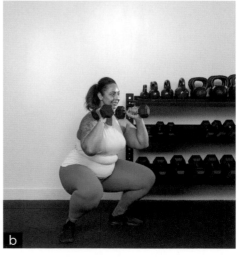

Figure 3.7 Front rack squat with two dumbbells: *(a)* starting position; *(b)* squat.

Single-Arm Front Rack Squat

Perform the single-arm front rack squat the same way as the front rack squat, only while holding one kettlebell on the outside of your wrist, again holding your chest tall (figure 3.8). Hold the weight at your chest with the other arm extended out in front of you. Stand with the feet hip-distance apart, toes turned out about 30 degrees. Drive your hips back and knees out. As you are sitting into your squat, focus on keeping your chest up so that the weight in your hand does not pull you forward. Just like in the front rack squat, when a heavy weight is put in front of the body, it wants to pull us down and forward. Even though we are adding weight on one side of the body, we are not adding an element of rotation to the mix. Place your free arm out to the side and hold it really strong. This helps create tension so that the weight doesn't pull you out of alignment.

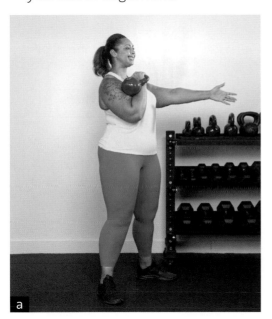
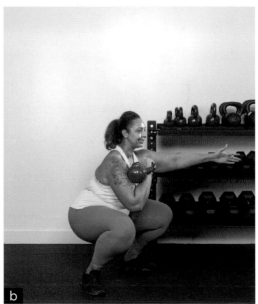

Figure 3.8   Single-arm front rack squat: *(a)* starting position; *(b)* squat.

Barbell Squat

It's time to use the squat rack (see Using a Squat Rack on page 38). A squat rack allows you to get into a safe and strong position with a bar on your back. It's not absolutely necessary to use a squat rack or a barbell, but it allows you to use more weight since dumbbells and kettlebells have lower limits. When you are setting up for a barbell squat, place the J-hooks (the pieces that the barbell is resting on) just below shoulder height. Most barbells have knurling, lines cut into the metal. To set up for a barbell squat, place your thumbs on the knurling and then wrap your hands around the bar. With the feet together, pull yourself under the bar so that the bar rests on your shoulder blades. Stand up tall (figure 3.9a). To get into position away from the squat rack, step one foot straight back, step your other foot back and out to the side, and then step back again with your first foot at the width you want your squat to be (figure 3.9b). You should now be ready to squat, but if you need to adjust your feet, go for it. With the bar on your back and your chest up tall, begin your squat: Drive your hips back and your knees out until you find depth (figure 3.9c). Keep tension throughout your body, and then stand up. The big difference a barbell squat has from a bodyweight, kettlebell, or dumbbell squat is where the weight sits. Our center of gravity shifts, and we have to work to keep ourselves balanced.

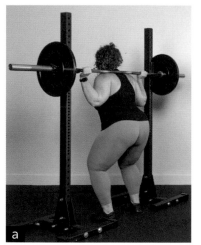 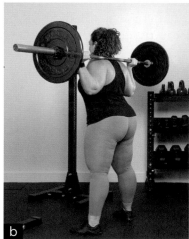 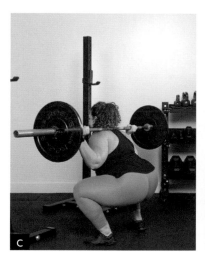

Figure 3.9 Barbell squat: *(a)* rack position; *(b)* starting position; *(c)* squat.

Deadlift

A deadlift is an efficient and safe way to pick something heavy off the floor. We must work to use our legs and core, keeping the weight as close to the body as possible. In a deadlift, we bend over and pick up a weight. It seems so simple, but remember the goal is to lift a lot of weight without getting hurt and to do it efficiently.

Deadlifting is one of the most efficient ways to gain strength in nearly every muscle in your body at once. You can lift the most weight with the deadlift, which is also empowering. I love being able to say I can deadlift 400 pounds. Just like the squat, it takes time and respect for your body and the movement to get there. Some people are naturally strong and able to pick up a lot of weight without thinking about it. Others, like me, have gone through the ringer and back to reach our goals.

Muscles

Primary: Gluteus maximus, hamstrings, latissimus dorsi

Secondary: Calves, rectus abdominis, obliques, erector spinae, quadriceps, adductors, rhomboids, trapezius

Instructions

Place your feet about hip-width apart, with the toes forward or slightly turned out. Hinge at the hips and push your hips back with a slight bend in your knees as you reach down to grab your equipment (figure 3.10a). This is the basic description of any deadlift—barbell, kettlebell,

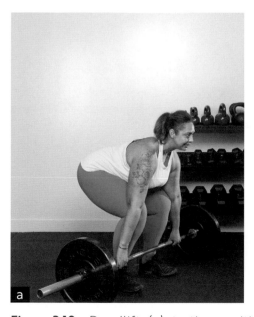
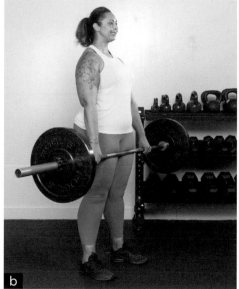

Figure 3.10   Deadlift: *(a)* starting position; *(b)* top position.

or dumbbell. You should have your equipment set up directly underneath you. At this point, your upper body should be nearly parallel to the floor. Check that your shoulders are away from your ears. Engage your back and create tension throughout the body. Lift the chest, take a deep breath in, and then stand straight up (figure 3.10*b*). Never drop your weight unless it's ripping the skin off of your hands. If the bar sits in your hands wrong or there is just a lot of weight and the bar rips the skin off of your hands, that would be an acceptable time to drop the bar. Once you are at full extension (standing straight up), it's time to hinge your hips, drive your butt back, slightly bend your knees, and bring the weight to the ground. Remember the term is *deadlift*; there should be a full stop on the ground, with a moment to reset, create tension, take that deep breath, and lift again.

Movement Focus

A common issue exercisers experience when doing a deadlift is rounding the back. I use the word *tension* a lot, and in order to lift a lot of weight, you must create tension. To prevent the lower back from rounding, which is a sign you are no longer under tension, you have to keep your hamstrings, glutes, core, and lats all active and engaged. It is easier said than done, but with practice you will understand what I mean—and get stronger.

Cues

- Stand with the feet hip-width apart.
- Hinge at the hips.
- Keep your upper body parallel to the floor.
- Slightly bend your knees.
- Create tension throughout the body.
- Straighten your arms.

Tips and Tricks

The sumo stance is probably the most comfortable stance to start with for some body types. The sumo creates room for your belly when you are bent over. In a traditional deadlift, the legs are kept pretty close together and you pick up the weight from the ground. The issue for people of size is that there isn't anywhere for that size to go. Sumo stance is a nice, wide stance. You can bring your legs out wide but still feel strong. Turn your toes out to the sides and drive your knees out so that when you bend over to pick up the weight, you have lots of room for your body. We will go into more detail about the sumo deadlift on page 57.

Variations

Kettlebell Deadlift Off a Block

Place the block directly between your feet with the kettlebell on top. Use a block that raises the kettlebell to the appropriate height for you. If you have a hard time reaching the kettlebell when you attempt the deadlift, try raising the height of the block. With the block, you won't have to bring yourself low to the ground to reach the weight. Load the hips, tighten the chest, take a deep breath in, and stand up (figure 3.11).

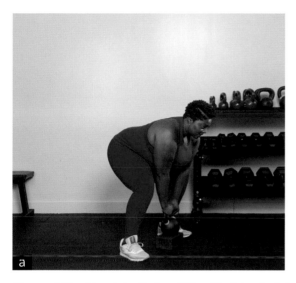 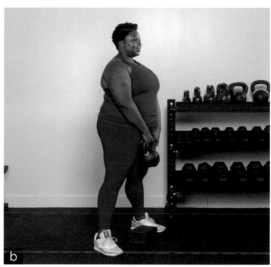

Figure 3.11 Kettlebell deadlift off a block: *(a)* starting position; *(b)* top position.

Kettlebell Deadlift From the Floor

Rather than lifting the kettlebell off a block, you are now just picking up the weight from the floor (figure 3.12). Place your feet about hip-width apart, with the toes forward or slightly turned out. Hinge at your hips and push your hips back with a slight bend in your knees as you reach down to grab your kettlebell. In order to get lower to the floor, you need to have more of a bend in your knees.

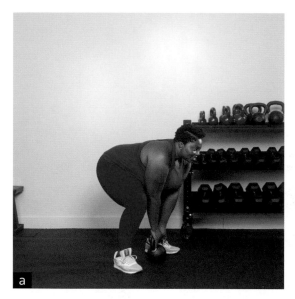
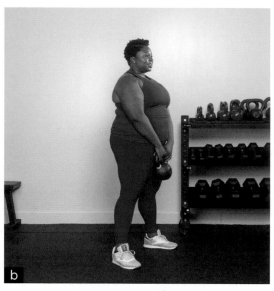

Figure 3.12 Kettlebell deadlift from the floor: *(a)* starting position; *(b)* lift.

Single-Arm Kettlebell Deadlift

The setup is the same as for the kettlebell deadlift from the floor. However, this time you are going to lift with only one arm (figure 3.13). Place your feet about hip-width apart, with the toes forward or slightly turned out. Hinge at your hips and push your hips back with a slight bend in your knees as you reach down to grab your kettlebell with one arm. Place the free arm out to the side and create tension. This helps you stay in alignment. When we only have a weight on one side of the body, it wants to pull us out of alignment. The challenge here is to use the core to keep that from happening.

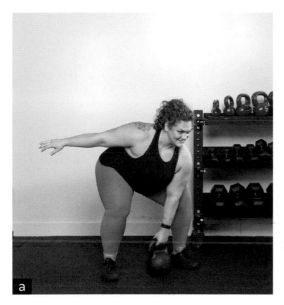
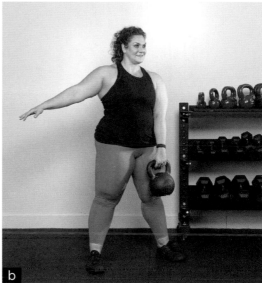

Figure 3.13 Single-arm kettlebell deadlift: *(a)* starting position; *(b)* lift.

Kettlebell or Dumbbell Suitcase Deadlift

A suitcase deadlift is applicable to everyday life. If you have ever had to carry heavy grocery bags in both hands, you have done a movement similar to this before. With the feet hip-width apart or a tad narrower and the weights sitting right outside the feet, drive your hips back, place your hands on each weight, and lift your chest (figure 3.14*a*). Check to make sure you create tension, then take that deep breath in and stand up (figure 3.14*b*). The weights stay outside the body. As you lower, drive your hips back and unlock your knees to set the kettlebells or dumbbells back on the floor. An easy way to check in with yourself about keeping your lats under tension for this movement is that if the weights hit your toes on the way down, you have let your chest collapse.

Using kettlebells makes it easier to find the floor than using dumbbells. If you are using dumbbells and are having trouble reaching the floor, either don't aim to hit the ground or place blocks by your sides and aim to hit the blocks.

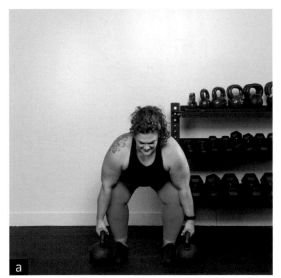 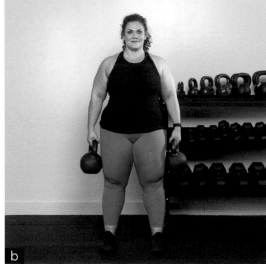

Figure 3.14 Kettlebell suitcase deadlift: *(a)* starting position; *(b)* top position.

Staggered Stance Deadlift

The staggered stance deadlift can be done with or without weight with one or two dumbbells. Standing tall, with the feet hip-width apart, step one foot back, about a foot behind and to the side (figure 3.15*a*). Stay on the ball of your back foot. Hinge your hips back, just as you would with the other deadlift movements (figure 3.15*b*). This time, there are a few things to focus on: (1) both knees should be slightly bent; (2) focus on finding the stretch in the hamstring on the front leg; and (3) keep your chest tall with the weight, if you use any, as close to the legs as possible. Hinge only to the point of feeling the stretch or barely below the knees, and then stand back up.

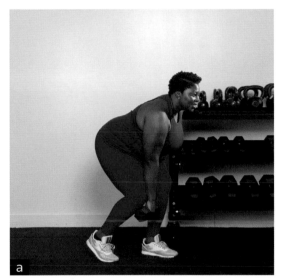 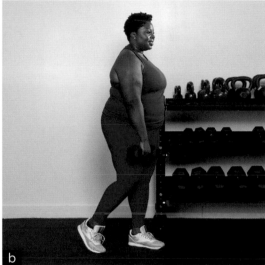

Figure 3.15 Staggered stance deadlift: (*a*) staggered stance; (*b*) hinge at the hips.

Single-Leg Deadlift

A single-leg deadlift (figure 3.16) is the same as a staggered stance deadlift except that your back leg is no longer on the floor. The focus here is on keeping your hips squared to the floor and maintaining stability. I highly recommend holding on to something sturdy when performing the single-leg deadlift, especially when you first start. Remember to keep your chest tall and, if you use weights, keep them close to the body. Standing on one leg, with your free leg bent to about 90 degrees, hinge your hips and drive your butt back. As you extend your free leg behind you, focus on the hips and driving your weight back.

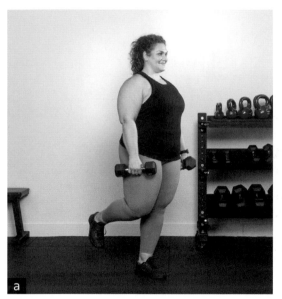 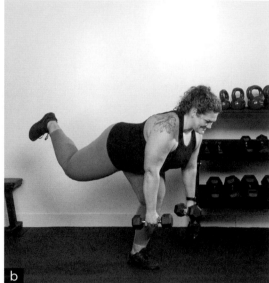

Figure 3.16 Single-leg deadlift: *(a)* staggered stance with back leg elevated; *(b)* hinge at the hips.

Hex Bar Deadlift

A hex bar is a bar in the shape of a hexagon. The handles are on the sides, and you step into the middle to use it. The hex bar deadlift (figure 3.17) is like a suitcase deadlift, but you can add more weight than you could using kettlebells or dumbbells. The setup to use a hex bar is the same setup as a kettlebell suitcase deadlift, except you don't need to worry about spacing the weights since the hex bar has them in a fixed location. A hex bar allows you to lift more weight and is also higher off the floor. If you are struggling to get in a good starting squat position due to the depth required, a hex bar is a great way to work on it. Place weights on the hex bar and step inside the bar. Make sure the handles are in line with your legs. Drive your hips back and slightly bend your knees as you grab the handles. Take a deep breath, create tension in your lats with a proud and tall chest, and stand up. Drive your hips back, slightly bending your knees, and find the floor to return.

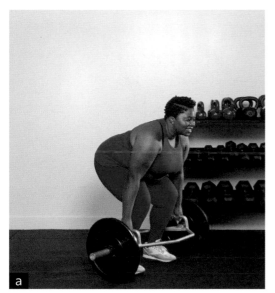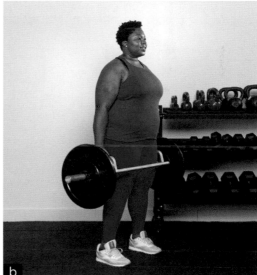

Figure 3.17 Hex bar deadlift: (a) starting position; (b) top position.

Straight Bar Deadlift

Step up to the bar with the feet hip-distance apart or narrower. Drive your hips back and slightly bend your knees so you can place your thumbs at the knurling on the bar and wrap your hands around the bar. Check in with your body to make sure your back is flat, your chest is up, and your muscles are under tension (figure 3.18a). Stand up by driving your feet into the floor and keeping your core tight (figure 3.18b). Stand tall but do not overextend; don't lean too far back. When you try to stand up taller, you might end up leaning into your lower back. Slowly drive your hips back and slightly bend your knees as you bring the weight back to the ground.

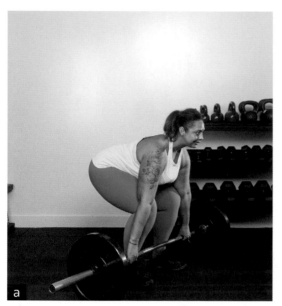 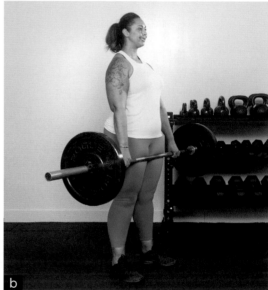

Figure 3.18 Straight bar deadlift: (a) starting position; (b) top position.

Sumo Deadlift

A sumo deadlift can be done with a straight bar (figure 3.19) or a kettle-bell, the major difference being the width of your stance. There is no right or wrong answer to how wide you stand, but the idea is that you are trying to get your body lower to the ground so that you don't have as far to lift the weight. Whether using a straight bar or kettlebell, place your arms inside your legs. Stand with the bar in front of you. Drive your hips back and knees out to the sides. With straight arms and tension in your lats, grab the bar. Take a deep breath, and drive your feet into the ground. Keep driving your knees out to the sides and stand up tall. Once at the top, slowly drive your hips back and slightly bend the knees to find the floor again.

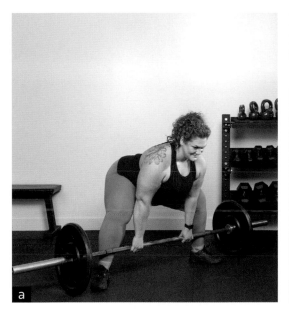 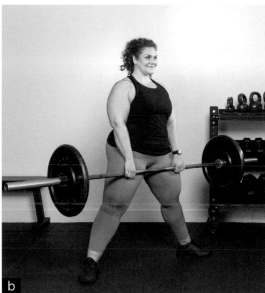

Figure 3.19 Sumo deadlift with a straight bar: (*a*) starting position; (*b*) top position.

Lunge

The best and easiest way I know to teach someone to do a lunge is to start from a standing position and ask them to come down to one knee. This is obviously not going to create the perfect lunge, but it helps in learning the movement. I have joked in the past that a lunge is like getting into a proposal position, getting down on one knee. It is taking a knee in sports; a lunge is used all the time. From what I have seen, the big issue for people when doing lunges is their knees. An improperly done lunge can place a lot of force on the knees. It might seem like a lunge isn't something that we use as often as a squat (sitting down) or a deadlift (picking things up), but we need to be able to get off the ground. It's inevitable that we will be on the ground at some point in our lives, whether it be because we decided to sit on the floor or because we fell. What if you find nothing or no one around to help you back up? More than likely, you will use some variation of a lunge to return to a standing position.

Muscles

Primary: Gluteus maximus, quadriceps

Secondary: Hamstrings, adductors

Instructions

Starting from the floor, get into a half kneeling position (proposal position; figure 3.20a). Make sure that you feel stable, hips are squared off, and your chest is up. Curl the back toes under, take a deep breath, drive your feet into the ground, and stand (figure 3.20b). From the top, instead of just dropping to the ground, think about sitting back as you do when you squat. Drive your hips back, keeping your weight off of your knees and in your glutes.

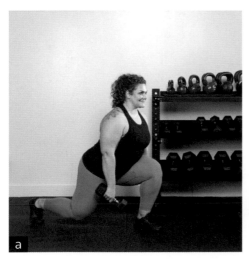
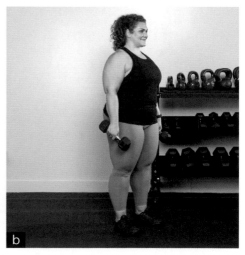

Figure 3.20 Lunge: (a) starting position; (b) top position.

Movement Focus

Let's bring our attention to the glutes versus the knees; this cue has worked for me for years to help people who have knee pain while lunging. Let's work on keeping the core stable. Often when we are lunging, we forget that the rest of our body matters. Put your focus into your hips and glutes, but also be sure that you are keeping your core strong. I often see that people's heels aren't on the ground. Pressing through the floor is the connection we have to creating strength. Be sure to push those feet into the ground! I also sometimes see the knees buckling in just like in a squat. The cue to drive your knees out applies to lunges as well.

Cues

- Drive your hips back.
- Feel the weight in your glutes.
- Hold your chest up.

Knees Passing the Toes

Knees passing the toes—it is one of fitness's biggest myths. In natural movements patterns, our knees will pass our toes because that is how the body works. Yet many people believe that this is wrong because they have pain when their knees pass over their toes.

There are a couple of reasons for this. The first involves general mobility of the knees, hips, and ankles. If you are lacking mobility in these joints, then you will likely feel some version of discomfort when you are pushing into a range of motion that the body isn't yet ready for. The second involves doing the movement correctly. Whether we are squatting, deadlifting, or lunging, we need to press through the floor with the entirety of the foot. What can happen, usually in a squat or lunge, is that the heels come off the ground and all of our weight gets pushed into the knees versus into the hips. This can put a lot of pressure on the knee joint.

Many fitness professionals believe that over time, if we keep letting our knees go over our toes when under load, we will cause damage to the joints. Yet this is the opposite of what these experts also believe, which is that we need to load the body to create strong bones and joints. At the end of the day, we need to try and move, do the squat or lunge that is best for our bodies, and trust what we believe to be right.

Variations

Split Squat

A split squat is also called a static lunge. Stand with your feet staggered, hip-distance apart (figure 3.21*a*). Drive your hips back, lowering your back knee toward the floor (figure 3.21*b*). With a full range of motion, your knee lightly touches the ground. Drive your feet through the floor and come back to the top.

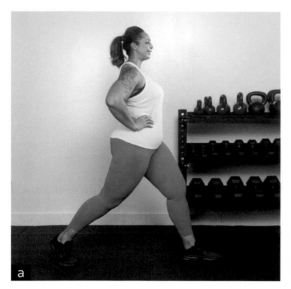
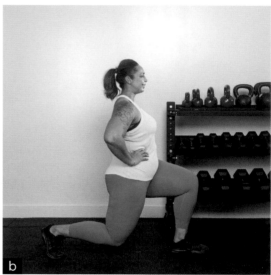

Figure 3.21   Split squat: *(a)* starting position; *(b)* bottom position.

Tips and Tricks

If bringing your knee all the way to the ground is too hard, place a yoga block under the knee. Working on range of motion to get to the ground takes time. You can also hold on to something like a bar or a TRX suspension system to help you ease toward the ground.

Backward Lunge

Stand with your feet together (figure 3.22a). Step back onto the ball of your foot. Try to keep your feet hip-distance apart. If your stance is too narrow, you lose a good base of support and can become unstable. As you are stepping back, drive your hips back and bend your back knee, bringing it toward the floor (figure 3.22b). Kiss the floor with your knee and then drive through your back foot and front foot to come back to a standing position with feet together.

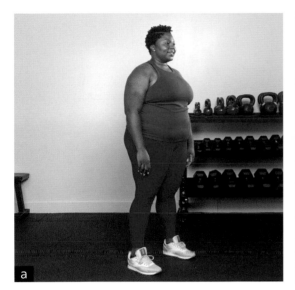
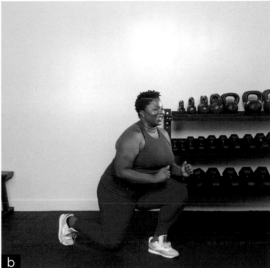

Figure 3.22 Backward lunge: (a) starting position; (b) bottom position.

> ### Tips and Tricks
>
> For the backward and forward lunges, your back foot is always the foot that is bent. The front foot always stays flat on the floor and drives into the ground.

Forward Lunge

Stand with your feet together (figure 3.23a). Take a step forward, again working to keep your feet hip-distance apart. As you step forward, lower your body toward the floor by bending your knees (figure 3.23b). Keep your weight in your hips and not your knees. Kiss the floor with your back knee and then drive through the floor to come back up. A big mistake that can happen with a front lunge is stepping too far forward and having a hard time coming back to the standing position. Be sure that your front foot is planted firmly on the ground and that you aren't on your toes.

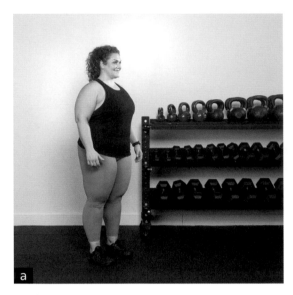 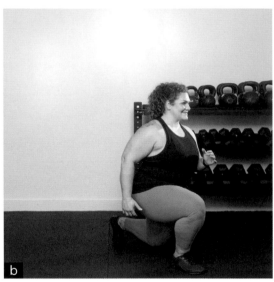

Figure 3.23 Forward lunge: *(a)* starting position; *(b)* bottom position.

Lateral Lunge

Stand with your feet together (figure 3.24*a*) and step out to the side (laterally). As you step to the side, drive your hips back and bend the knee on the side you're stepping to (figure 3.24*b*). A couple of things to pay attention to: Your knee should be in line with your toes, so work to sit back with your knee and toes facing forward. Your other leg should stay straight. Don't step out too far because this can uncomfortably stretch the inner thigh. Once you have found your lunge position, drive into the ground and push off the floor to come back to standing.

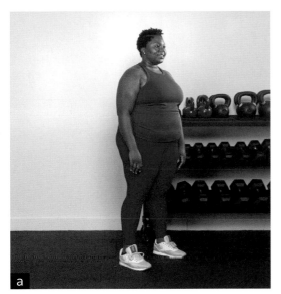 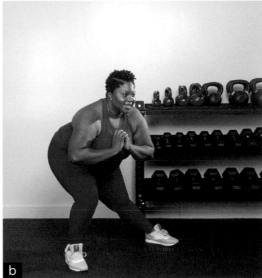

Figure 3.24 Lateral lunge: *(a)* starting position; *(b)* step to the side.

Step-Up

Most people do step-ups every day. Have you ever walked up a flight of stairs? Technically speaking, step-ups are the easiest hip hinge there is because there is less range of motion needed for step-ups than for other exercises like the deadlift. However, step-ups are an incredible unilateral leg exercise, providing a way to work on single-leg strength and improve imbalances. Often people think of step-ups as a cardio exercise. As a cardio exercise, it's usually done rather quickly and without focus. While there is a time and a place for cardio step-ups, working on step-ups with control is super important and can be very difficult. Unilateral strength not only makes you stronger but can also help the body improve imbalances that may cause pain. If you notice one side is truly weaker than the other, it is okay to do extra sets on that side, to put your focus into that side and work to make it stronger.

Muscles

Primary: Quadriceps

Secondary: Gluteus maximus, hamstrings

Instructions

Stand in front of a step or stable box. Start with a low box, and then with time and progress, use a higher box. Begin by placing one foot on top of the box (figure 3.25a). Step up by pressing through that foot to lift yourself to the top of the box (figure 3.25b). Hinge at your hips and bend your top knee to slowly lower yourself back to the ground.

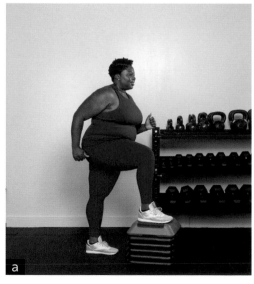
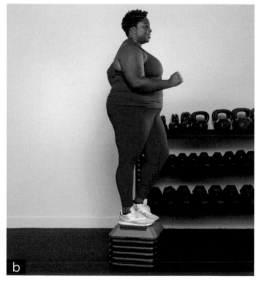

Figure 3.25 Step-up: (a) starting position with foot on box; (b) top position.

Movement Focus

Step-ups can be done quickly or slowly. When aiming for strength and stability, it is best to do step-ups slowly, under control. Focus on the leg on the box, both when stepping up and when stepping back down. If you push off the floor with the foot that's on the ground, that won't help you to develop strength in the leg on the box. On your way down, make it count. Maintain control by keeping your weight in the leg on the box; don't just drop back to the floor. A helpful tip is to create tension in your arms, either keeping them by your sides or holding them out in front of you. This helps stabilize you.

Cues

- Drive through the foot on the box.
- Hinge at the hips.
- Keep your weight in the leg on the box.

Variations

Dumbbell Step-Up

The movement doesn't change; we just add some weight. Holding the dumbbells may help you to feel more stable because your arms are forced into creating tension. Be careful not to react to the added weight by launching yourself off the floor with the bottom leg. Stand in front of a step or stable box with a dumbbell in each hand. Place one foot on top of the box (figure 3.26*a*). Step up by pressing through the foot on the box, lifting yourself to the top of the box (figure 3.26*b*). Hinge at your hips and bend your top knee to slowly lower yourself back to the ground.

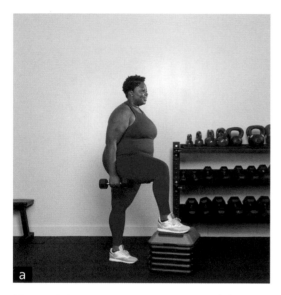
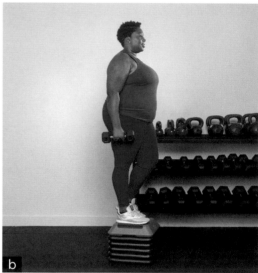

Figure 3.26 Dumbbell step-up: *(a)* starting position; *(b)* top position.

Step Down

The main difference with a step-down is you start from the top of the box. Stand with both feet on the box (figure 3.27a). Lift one foot off the box, hinge your hips back, and very slowly lower the foot toward the ground (figure 3.27b). Don't rest on the floor; just lightly tap the floor with your toe, then drive up with the leg that's on top of the box. You can perform the step-down with or without dumbbells.

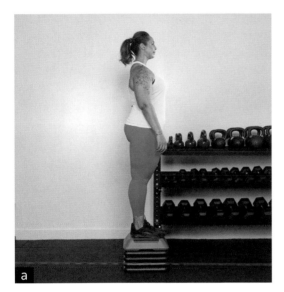 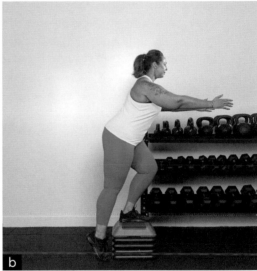

Figure 3.27 Step-down: *(a)* starting position; *(b)* foot lightly taps the floor.

CONCLUSION

Our legs hold us up. They help us get from place to place, sit down, and stand up. All the exercises in this chapter help strengthen the lower half of your body. There are variations and ways to work with the basic movements that our bodies can do. Start slowly with light weight and work your way up. Remember that if something feels wrong, it probably is, so take your time and reset. Remember that even though the focus of each exercise in this chapter is to work the legs, the core must be involved in order for you to execute them properly. For bodies of size, range of motion can be hard to achieve in the beginning, but with time, practice, and strength, you will get there. I like to remind my clients that we don't train to lift—we train for everyday life. When you get up from a chair, use your legs, hold your belly strong, push through the floor, and stand up tall. Relate your workouts to everyday life and get your repetitions wherever you can.

PUSH
AND PULL

Body strength doesn't come as easily to women as it does to men, so what that tells me is that we are going to have to work harder for it. I like to prove people wrong. I'm a 260-pound woman, and I can do a set of 20 unbroken push-ups. I like to be just as strong as, if not stronger than, the boys.

This chapter is all about upper-body strength. Upper-body strength isn't just about being able to do push-ups. It's about being able to do things in everyday life on your own: put the luggage in the overhead bin, carry the laundry up the stairs, carry your groceries out from the store, or even get yourself off the ground. In chapter 3, we learned how lower-body strength is important for movements such as getting off the floor, but sometimes we need a little help from the upper body. We need to push or pull ourselves up.

The upper body (figure 4.1) features some of the most important muscles in movement, flexibility, and strength. The exercises in this chapter work the muscles of the chest, shoulders, arms, and back.

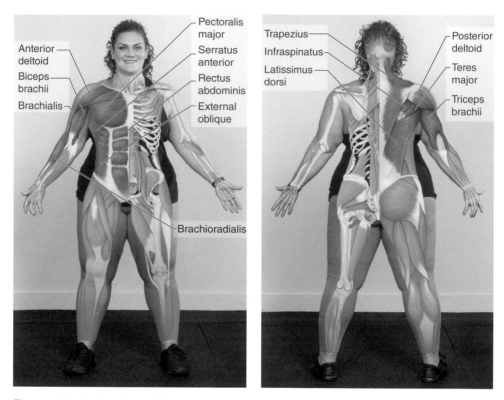

Figure 4.1   Muscles of the upper body.

Push-Up

Light as a feather, stiff as a board. A push-up works only if you can keep your body and muscles tight so that they can all work and move together.

Muscles

Primary: Pectoralis, triceps, anterior deltoid

Secondary: Biceps, rectus abdominis, obliques, quadriceps, erector spinae

Instructions

From a plank position (page 107), squeeze your thighs and your butt, and hold your abdomen strong (figure 4.2a). To begin lowering yourself, I want you to think about pulling your shoulder blades together. Be sure to bring your chest and abdomen down at the same time (figure 4.2b). Once you've hit full range of motion, which means chest to the ground (no resting!), push through the floor with your hands and feet and drive straight back up. There are many variations of push-ups, but the idea is to use your upper body and core strength to get up off the floor.

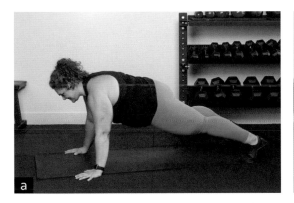 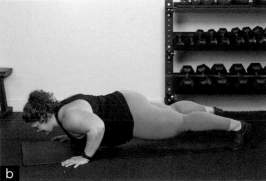

Figure 4.2 Push-up: (a) top position; (b) bottom position.

Movement Focus

Taking the time to focus on how to hold our body in a strong position greatly benefits all the movements we do. A common problem is the abdomen sags down to the ground, which means you are not engaging the muscles in the core. This is where it is the most obvious that the push-up isn't just an upper-body exercise. If you find that your abdomen sags, squeeze your butt and almost slightly round your lower back up toward the ceiling.

I sometimes also see the elbows flaring and the shoulders hiked up to the neck. These two issues tend to go hand in hand. When the elbows flare, you are probably elevating the shoulder blades, which leads to a weaker position in your push-up. Once in plank, be sure to check that your shoulders are down and away from your ears. When lowering in the push-up, your elbows should be angled back at about 45 degrees.

Cues

- Pull your chest to the ground.
- Engage the core muscles.
- Squeeze the glutes.
- Push through the floor.

Variations

Hands Elevated Push-Up

Let's start at the wall and work our way down. Start a push-up progression against a wall (figure 4.3), then move to a countertop, to a chair, and then closer and closer to the ground. The more your upper body is elevated, the easier the push-up is. In a gym setting, you can use a squat rack or a Smith machine (normally used for squats) for push-ups (figure 4.4). A squat rack or Smith machine can be lowered inch by inch, usually numbered, so you can easily measure progress on your elevated push-ups. As you get stronger, you can lower the bar and do push-ups one inch lower. Nothing changes in terms of how to do the push-up; the only thing you need to pay attention to is that you are working to keep your wrists under your shoulders.

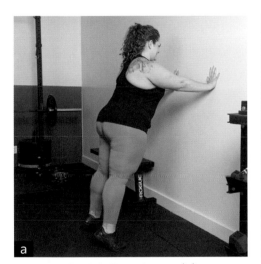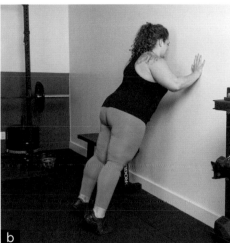

Figure 4.3   Wall push-up: *(a)* top position; *(b)* bottom position.

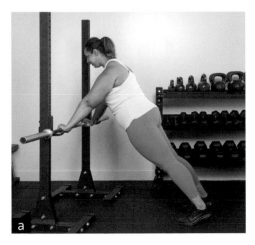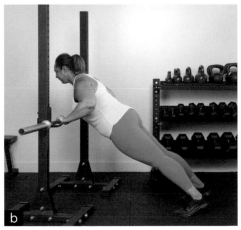

Figure 4.4   Smith machine (or squat rack) push-up: *(a)* top position; *(b)* bottom position.

Kneeling Push-Up

Starting from the plank position, drop your knees to the ground (figure 4.5a). Make sure you are still in plank position and not in an all-fours position; the knees should be slightly behind your hips. Lower to the bottom position (figure 4.5b) and push back up, keeping your body in a long line from the top of the head to the knees throughout the movement.

When performing kneeling push-ups, some people lose contact between their feet and the ground. Some people crisscross their lower legs. As I said in the setup, begin from a full plank position and maintain contact with the ground with your feet and knees. We create force and power by pushing through the ground, so push those feet into the ground as much as if your knees were not on the floor.

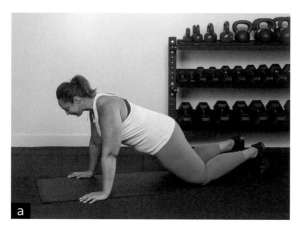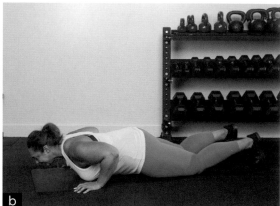

Figure 4.5 Kneeling push-up: (a) top position; (b) bottom position.

Negative Push-Up

Negative push-ups are a great way to work on strength. The objective is to control yourself in the eccentric phase, which means to lower yourself to the floor with control. Begin in your normal setup for a push-up or kneeling push-up. This time bring your whole body down to the floor as slowly as you can. Be sure your chest hits the floor before your abdomen (figure 4.6). The best part of the negative push-up is it doesn't matter how you get back up; just focus on the down.

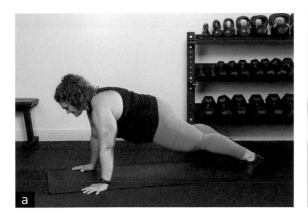 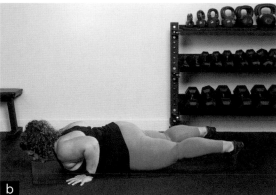

Figure 4.6 Negative push-up: *(a)* top position; *(b)* bottom position (chest hits the floor before the abdomen).

Chest Press

The chest (or bench) press is a great movement for building upper-body strength by adding weight in different variations, versus a push-up requiring you to lift your own body weight. Chest exercises like a chest press or chest fly also help you learn to brace the core. The bench press is one of your three powerlifting movements, along with the squat and the deadlift. As with all upper-body exercises, bench press is usually not as strong as lower-body movements. Using these movements can greatly improve that upper-body strength.

Muscles

Primary: Pectoralis, anterior deltoid, triceps
Secondary: Latissimus dorsi, glutes, rhomboids

Instructions

Sit on one end of a weight bench. Bring a set of dumbbells to your thighs. As you lie back onto the bench, bring the weights to your shoulders. Lie flat on your back, with your feet pressing into the ground (knees bent) to provide a strong base of support. Hold your elbows out to the sides of your chest. Make sure your shoulders are away from your ears and your elbows are at about 45 degrees (figure 4.7a). Focus on pressing your feet into the ground and using the power in your glutes as you press the weights up toward the ceiling (figure 4.7b). The arms should end in a locked-out position with the weights straight above your chest, not your face. Slowly pulling your shoulder blades together, bring your arms back to the start position.

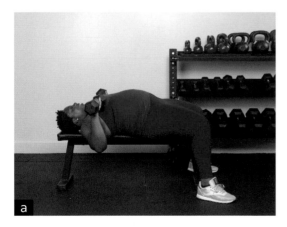 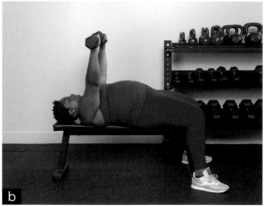

Figure 4.7   Chest press: *(a)* start position; *(b)* top position.

Movement Focus

It may seem simple enough to lie on your back and press some weight into the air. But it is also an opportunity to work on creating stability and tension in the body. When lying on your back, you may not think about needing to be stable, but if you want to be able to press a lot of weight, stability is a key factor in doing so. Try this drill I like to do with my clients. Grab a friend or stand by a wall. Stand up tall, put your arms out in the front of you, and make fists. Have your friend push against your fists; if your elbows bend, you aren't creating as much tension as possible or holding a stable position. If you don't have a friend available, press your knuckles into the wall and think about pushing through the wall as though you are going to make a hole. You should be able to feel how your whole body is working to create stability and tension in the shoulders. You can also test this while lying on your back. Hold the arms up straight in the air and make those fists. Have a friend press down on your fists and try to push your arms side to side. If you are using your whole body, it will be hard to move your arms at all.

Cues

- Pull the weight to your body.
- Press through the floor as you push the weight away from you.
- Use your legs and your whole body as you press.

Variations

Dumbbell Floor Chest Press

You begin this lift the same as the chest press on a bench, except this time your body is on the floor (figure 4.8). You get a little less range of motion because the floor stops your arms from going too far back, which makes it a great alternative that's gentler on your shoulders. The floor press requires you to use only upper-body strength because your lower body isn't involved in the push.

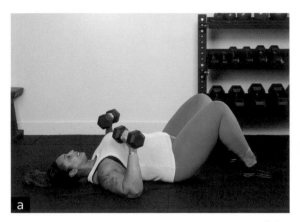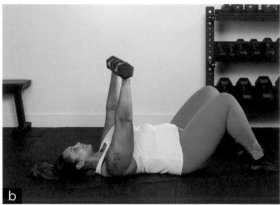

Figure 4.8 Dumbbell floor chest press: *(a)* start position; *(b)* press.

Dumbbell Chest Press on a Ball

This press sets up similarly to the press on a bench. Sit on a stability ball with the weights on your thighs. As you walk your feet forward, slowly let the ball roll to your back and bring the weights to your shoulders (figure 4.9). Your upper body rests on the stability ball as you do your chest press. Because of the unstable position, your core and lower body work to keep you in position as you press the weight up. You can adjust how far apart your feet are; the closer they are, the more difficult it is to keep your balance.

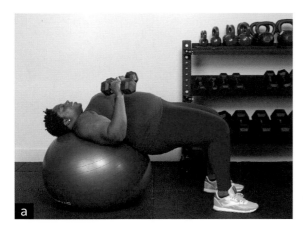 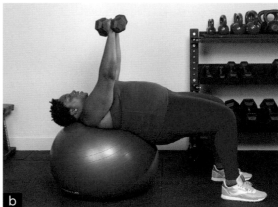

Figure 4.9 Dumbbell chest press on a ball: *(a)* start position; *(b)* press.

Dumbbell Chest Fly

Lying on a bench with a dumbbell in each hand, start with the arms straight up above the chest, palms facing each other (figure 4.10a). Slowly lower your arms outward, away from the midline of your body. Keep your arms almost straight, with a slight bend in the elbows, until you get to about 180 degrees (figure 4.10b). As you bring them back up, it should look as though you are hugging a tree. A chest fly is always done with less weight than a press because the farther a weight gets away from your body, the heavier it feels. This exercise can be done on the floor (knees bent or straight), on a bench, or on a ball.

To do a chest fly from a ball, start by sitting on an exercise ball with the weights on your thighs. Slowly walk your feet forward as you roll yourself down. Bring the weights to your chest. Your upper back and neck are relaxed on the ball. Bring your arms straight up above your chest. Before you start to lower the weight, check your hips and make sure that you are squeezing your butt and pushing your hips up toward the sky. Keep holding that strong core position as you do your chest fly repetitions.

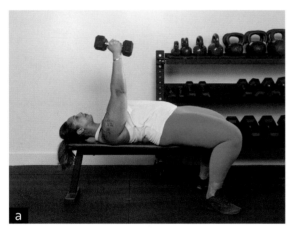 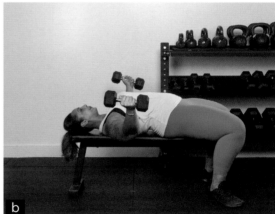

Figure 4.10 Dumbbell chest fly: (a) start position; (b) bottom position.

Barbell Bench Press

To perform this press safely, you need a rack with the rack set to the appropriate height (see Tips and Tricks). Lie with your back flat on the bench and your feet flat on the floor. (If you can't reach the floor, put plates or boxes under your feet.) Drive your knees out, like when you squat. Arch your lower back so that the only two parts of your body touching the bench are your butt and your upper back. Drive your shoulder blades together and into the bench. You should feel lots of tension created throughout the body in this position. Roll the bar to the end of the J-hook of the rack (away from the actual rack) and unrack the weight. Many people start their bench press from the rack, but this is incorrect. Wait until you have set your arms straight up above your chest and have taken a deep breath in to brace your core (figure 4.11a). Pull the barbell down to your chest (figure 4.11b) and then press it straight back up. I say pull the barbell down because you want to be in control of the weight; don't let it just fall to your chest. As the weight increases, it is very helpful to have a spotter or use a rack with safety bars.

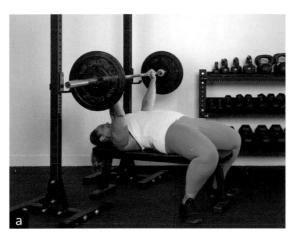 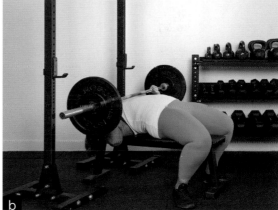

Figure 4.11 Barbell bench press: (a) start position; (b) bottom position.

Tips and Tricks

When you are lying with your back on the bench, put your arms straight up in the air. The bar height should be at about your wrists. Another important tip for when you are benching is not to clip the weights on to the bar. If for any reason you can't press the weight back up, you can dump the weights off to the sides. When we squat or deadlift, we usually clip so that we don't have weights that shift around. Weight shifting on the bar can happen when we bench press as well, but unless you have a spot, it's much safer to use an unclipped bar.

Row

We need to pull more than we push. We spend so much of our lives pushing or in positions that weaken our posterior chain (muscles on the back of our body). Old-school training worked on vanity muscles—the ones we could see in the mirror—forgetting about what helps us maintain good posture. The row is one of those good-posture exercises. The row, like every other exercise we are talking about, has a specific group of muscles it works. But if done properly and with intention, it can work others.

Muscles

Primary: Latissimus dorsi, posterior deltoid, rhomboids, teres major, trapezius

Secondary: Forearms and biceps (grip and some pulling), erector spinae, hamstrings, glutes (positioning)

Instructions

Stand with your knees slightly bent and core muscles engaged. Grab the handles of a cable machine or resistance band. The start position of the cable or the resistance band should be just below chest height, but it doesn't have to be perfect. Start with your arms straight as you pull your shoulders down away from your ears and keep your chest tall (figure 4.12a). Pull the handles closer to your chest, keeping your elbows close to your body (figure 4.12b). Don't overpull; you don't want to pull so far that your shoulders start to round forward. You also want to keep your wrists neutral throughout the movement; no need to try to pull farther by rounding your wrists into the body.

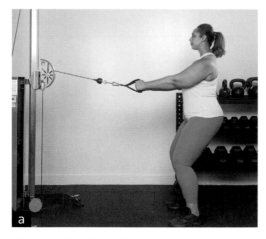 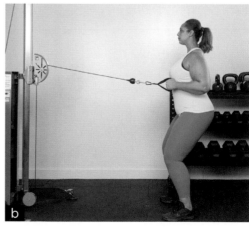

Figure 4.12 Standing cable machine row: *(a)* start position; *(b)* bent-arm position.

Movement Focus

Pull your shoulders up to your ears. This is where we generally live; I'm having you be more dramatic about it. Now, pull your shoulders as far down from your ears as possible and pull them back so you are opening your chest. This is a strong, confident position to be in, and pulling movements help us to practice this position. The row movement itself is simple. We are pulling a weight closer to our bodies. The pull is the easy part; it is keeping the body in the right position that can be difficult. Like I said, we tend to default to a shoulders elevated and forward position, so as our muscles fatigue, they tend to go back to what has been ingrained in our minds and muscle memory.

Cues

- Bring your shoulders down and back, away from your ears.
- Keep your chest tall.

Variations

Standing Single-Arm Row

Row with one arm at a time (figure 4.13). It's a great way to focus on not overpulling and rotating in the core. Let this movement become an anti-rotation or a core-stabilizing exercise.

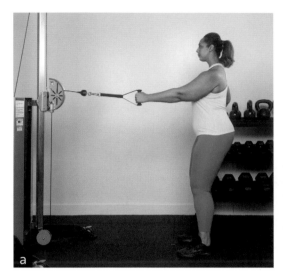 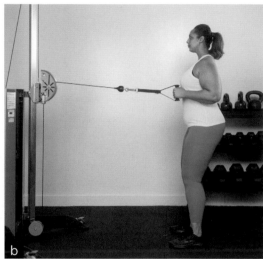

Figure 4.13 Standing single-arm row: *(a)* start position; *(b)* bent-arm position.

Half Kneeling Single-Arm Row

The pull stays the same. From a half kneeling position, pull with the arm that is on the same side as the knee on the ground (figure 4.14). So, if your left knee is on the floor, you are pulling with your left arm.

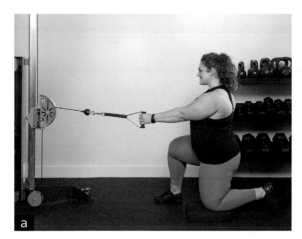 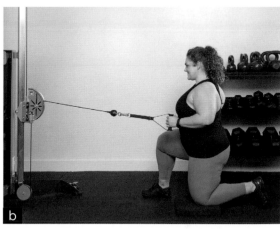

Figure 4.14 Half kneeling single-arm row: (*a*) start position; (*b*) bent-arm position.

Single-Arm Row*

Begin with the left knee and left palm on a weight bench (figure 4.15a). Slightly bend the right leg. Back is flat. The right hand pulls the weight to your chest (figure 4.15b). Again, the pulling motion is the same, but it is coming from below you instead of in front. Gravity plays a part, so once you have brought the weight to the top, pause, then slowly release back down, keeping your shoulder on tension. Don't let the weight pull you down.

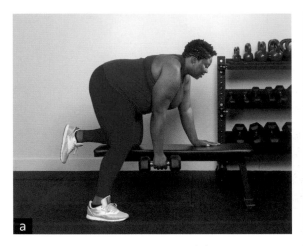 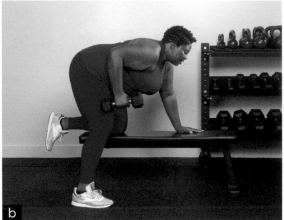

Figure 4.15 Single-arm row: *(a)* start position; *(b)* top position.

The movements marked with an * can be done with a dumbbell (DB) or kettlebell (KB).

Three-Point Stance Single-Arm Row*

Place one hand on a weight bench. The back is flat and the feet are about hip-width apart. Grip the weight in your other hand. Pull the weight to your body (figure 4.16) and slowly release back down.

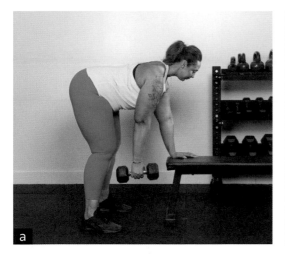 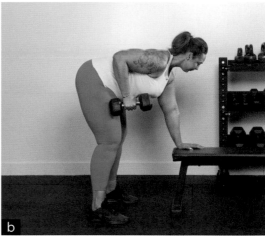

Figure 4.16   Three-point stance single-arm row: (a) start position; (b) top position.

Dual Bent-Over Row*

Standing tall with a dumbbell in each hand, hinge your hips back with slightly bent knees (figure 4.17a). (This might feel similar to deadlifting.) With your shoulders on tension, pull the weight up to your body (figure 4.17b) and slowly lower back down. Be mindful of your lower back in this position; be sure to keep it flat.

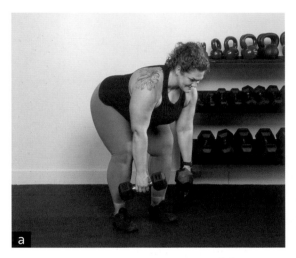 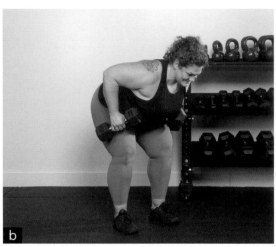

Figure 4.17 Dual bent-over row: *(a)* start position; *(b)* top position.

Single-Arm Bent-Over Row*

This is performed like a dual bent-over row, except you only do one arm at a time (figure 4.18). The main difference is you are working on anti-rotation of the body and not letting the weight pull you over since you are only holding one weight.

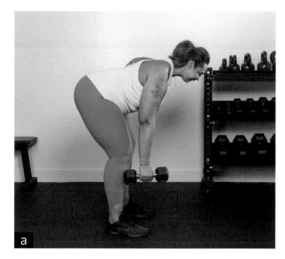 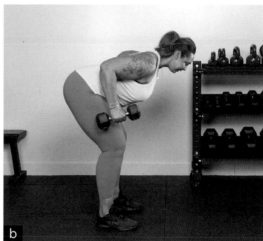

Figure 4.18   Single-arm bent-over row: *(a)* start position; *(b)* top position.

Barbell Bent-Over Row (Pronated or Supinated)

With a barbell in both hands and arms straight, hinge forward at your hips and slightly bend your knees (figure 4.19a). With a flat back and chest lifted, pull the barbell to your chest, about where your bra line would be (figure 4.19b). Slowly release the weight toward your legs until your arms are straight again, being sure not to let the bar get too far away from you. As with a deadlift, holding the bar away from you can cause your lower back to round and risk injury. Keep the bar close to your body at all times.

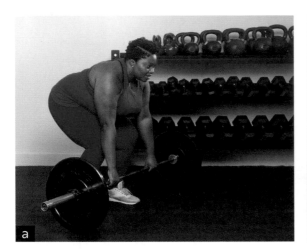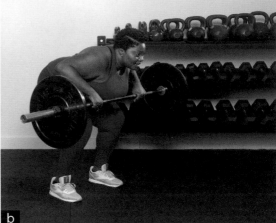

Figure 4.19   Barbell bent-over row: *(a)* bottom position; *(b)* top position.

Tips and Tricks

Pronated grip on a barbell row is when the palms face the body (figure 4.20). Supinated grip on a barbell row is when the palms face away from the body (figure 4.21). It's an underhand grip.

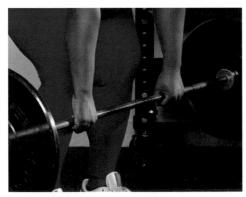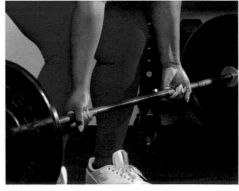

Figure 4.20   Pronated grip.   **Figure 4.21**   Supinated grip.

Band Pull-Apart

Begin by holding the ends of a resistance band in each hand with your arms straight out in front of you and palms facing the floor (figure 4.22a). Keeping your arms straight, pull your shoulder blades together as you pull the band apart (figure 4.22b). Slowly release back to the start position. Work to keep your shoulders away from your ears; it's easy to hike your shoulders while doing this movement.

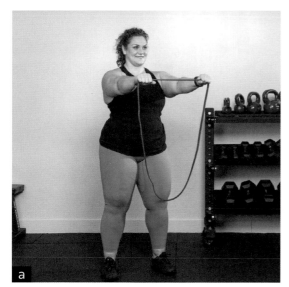 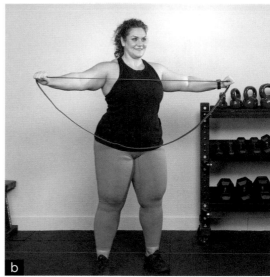

Figure 4.22 Band pull-apart: (a) start position; (b) open position.

Bent-Over Reverse Fly*

Stand with a weight in each hand. Hinge forward from your hips so that you are now in a bent-over position, similar to your bent-over row. With straight arms, pull your shoulders away from your ears and pull your shoulder blades together (figure 4.23a). Lift the weights up and out to each side so that they are in line with the shoulders (figure 4.23b). Slowly lower back down. Try not to use momentum.

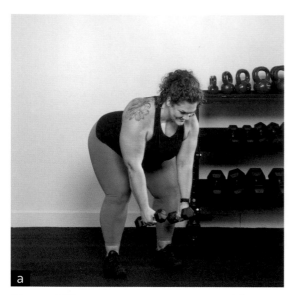 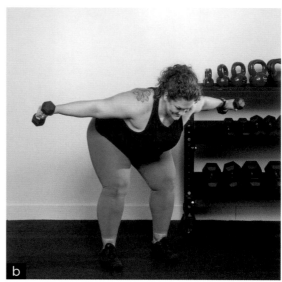

Figure 4.23 Bent-over reverse fly: (a) start position; (b) top position.

Pull-Down

The instructions for the exercises in this section are all very different, so we won't begin with one primary exercise. While the pull-down movements are each done differently, they primarily target the latissimus dorsi. Muscles in the shoulders, upper back, and upper arms are involved in several of these exercises, as well. Your lats are among the biggest muscles in your body and responsible for a lot of movements. Working on these muscles can help improve your posture and your deadlift. If you have the goal of being able to do a pull-up, you must work on your lat strength first.

Muscles

Primary: Latissimus dorsi, teres major

Secondary: Posterior deltoid, trapezius, rhomboids, levator scapulae, biceps, brachialis, brachioradialis, triceps, rotator cuff (supraspinatus, infraspinatus, teres minor, subscapularis)

Seated Lat Pull-Down

Using either a cable machine or resistance bands, sit on the bench seat or the floor with the chest lifted. For a lat pull-down, the cable or resistance band will be anchored above you. Grab the bar or band with your arms overhead and in a wide position (figure 4.24*a*). Lift your chest toward the ceiling and pull your shoulder blades down and away from your ears. It is okay to have a small arch in the lower back. Pull the weight straight down by bending your elbows (figure 4.24*b*); the bar should land at about your clavicle, and a band shouldn't go any lower than your armpits. Slowly release the weight back up, keeping your shoulders down and away from the ears with tension.

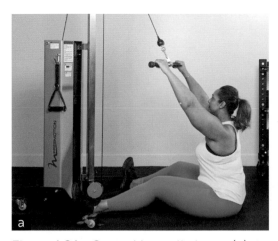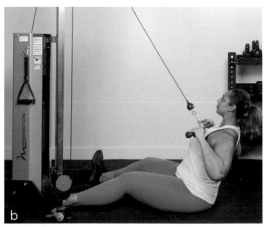

Figure 4.24   Seated lat pull-down: *(a)* start position; *(b)* bottom position.

Movement Focus

A seated lat pull-down is a fantastic way to work on back strength—and upper-body strength in general. If you want to be able to do pull-ups or a version of a pull-up, the lat pull-down should be your first step. Working on grip strength and back strength with the seated lat pull-down helps you with moves like the deadlift. One thing to make sure of when doing the lat pull-down is not to use too much momentum or lean too far back when pulling. A little bit of leaning back is okay because it helps you keep your chest open. Focusing on keeping your chest up and open is key. Otherwise, you may overpull at the bottom and cause your chest and shoulders to round forward, which isn't a safe or strong position for the shoulders.

Cues

■ Keep your chest up.

■ Think of pulling with your back muscles, not your arms.

Straight-Arm Pull-Down

Begin standing, with a wide grip either on a bar or band, handles or band anchored overhead (figure 4.25*a*). Slightly bend your knees, sit your hips back, and lift your chest. Keeping your arms straight or with a small bend in the elbows, pull the weight to your hip crease (figure 4.25*b*). Slowly release with the arms straight.

Movement Focus

The main difference that you feel with a straight-arm pull-down is more triceps and core work. When pulling the weight in toward your body, it almost feels as though you are doing crunches. I don't want you to actually crunch in, but you need to hold your core muscles really strong. Like a lat pull-down, if you overpull, your chest caves in and your shoulders round. So, we want to again focus on keeping the chest lifted and shoulders down.

Cues

- Straighten your arms.
- Lift your chest.

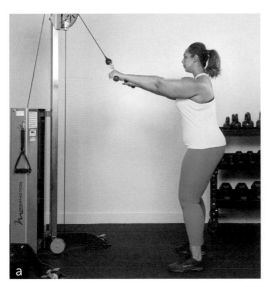 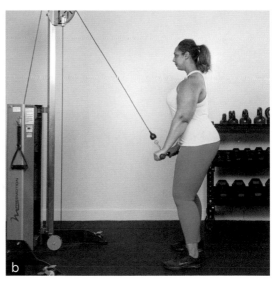

Figure 4.25 Straight-arm pull-down: *(a)* start position; *(b)* bottom position.

Dumbbell Pull-Over

While sitting on a weight bench, grab the very bottom of a dumbbell with your hands in a triangle shape. As you lie back on the bench, lift the weight straight up above your head. The weight should be positioned directly above your chest, with straight arms (figure 4.26a). Slowly lower the weight directly behind your head (figure 4.26b), as if you were going to set it on the floor behind you. Only go as far as you feel your shoulders can handle, and then slowly bring the weight back to the start position. It may be more comfortable to keep a slight bend in the elbows, and that's totally acceptable here.

Movement Focus

This is a lat-dominant movement, but because of the positioning of the body, triceps and core are involved. When lowering the weight behind your head, be aware that your lower back wants to come off the bench. It's okay if it raises off the bench a bit, but try to keep it down and only allow your arms to go back as far as your lower back and core stay strong.

Cues

- ■ Straighten your arms.
- ■ Keep your abdomen strong.

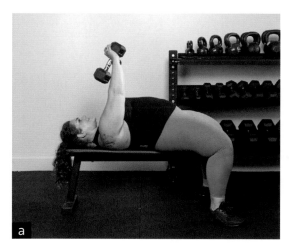 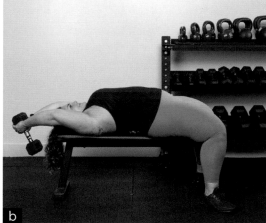

Figure 4.26 Dumbbell pull-over: (a) start position; (b) bottom position.

Overhead Press

The goal with all shoulder press movements is to get the weight straight up overhead. Each variation of the shoulder press changes slightly but can make a huge difference. Overhead pressing movements are as important for the health of the shoulder girdle as any other upper-body movements, but they can be harder when people lack overhead mobility. The shoulder joint is complex, and sometimes changing the variation of the shoulder movement can give you a greater ability to complete the movements and work on your strength.

Muscles

Each movement slightly changes which muscles are primary or secondary.

Primary: Deltoids (anterior, medial, posterior), pectoralis, upper trapezius, triceps

Secondary: Rotator cuff (supraspinatus, infraspinatus, teres minor, subscapularis)

Instructions

To perform an overhead press, start by standing, kneeling, or sitting with good posture and alignment of the body. When we stand for overhead movements, we use all the muscles in the body down to the feet. We have to work to press through the floor to create as much strength as possible. You can lift the most from a standing position. When we kneel, we are using our glutes and core, and our legs are no longer involved. When sitting, we have now taken the glutes and legs out of the equation and the main focus is on the core and shoulders. Hold a weight in each hand (figure 4.27a). Take a deep breath into your belly and press the weights up overhead (figure 4.27b). Your arms should be in line with your ears. Keep your ribcage pressed down, not flaring out. Slowly bring the weights back toward your shoulders.

Tips and Tricks

All of the overhead press movements can be done with resistance bands, dumbbells, or kettlebells.

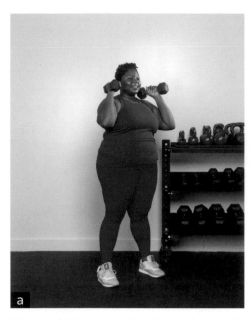 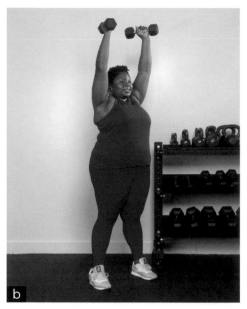

Figure 4.27 Dumbbell overhead shoulder press: *(a)* start position; *(b)* top position.

Movement Focus

Two major factors make the shoulder press one of the hardest movements: mobility and stability. We covered shoulder mobility in the section about overhead press and shoulder stability with the chest press. When pressing a weight above your head, you need mobility for alignment and stability for a strong position and control of the weight. Pressing the weight straight up isn't hard, but if you have mobility issues, it's hard to get your arms in line with your head. If you aren't in alignment, the weight feels heavier and pulls your shoulders into funny positions.

Cues

- Keep your arms in line with your ears.
- Keep your ribcage closed (i.e., don't let the ribcage flare open when your arms are straight overhead).

Variations

Military (Wide) Shoulder Press

With a dumbbell in each hand, place your arms in a wide position with your elbows at 90-degree angles, palms facing forward (figure 4.28*a*). Press your arms straight up above your head (figure 4.28*b*) and slowly lower them back to the original position.

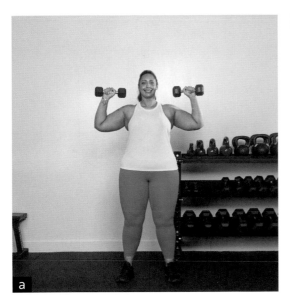
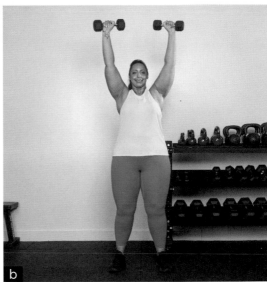

Figure 4.28 Military (wide) shoulder press: *(a)* start position; *(b)* top position.

Single-Arm Shoulder Press

Hold one dumbbell at your shoulder, palm facing inward (figure 4.29a). Press the dumbbell straight up in line with the ear (figure 4.29b), hold at the top for a moment, and slowly lower back to the start position.

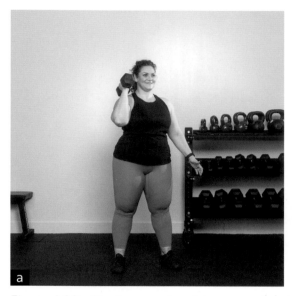 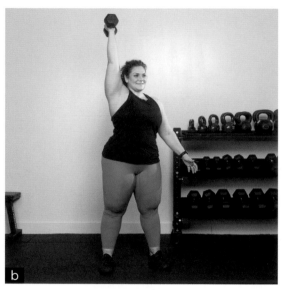

Figure 4.29   Single-arm shoulder press: (a) start position; (b) top position.

Barbell Overhead Press

Place your thumbs on the knurling of a barbell that's in a squat rack, and grip the barbell so that your palms are facing the floor. As you pull yourself under the barbell, your grip changes so that your palms are facing away from you (figure 4.30a). With the bar in your hands and resting on the collarbone, step out of the rack. Before you start your press, make sure you feel sturdy. With the bar at your collarbone, take a deep breath and brace before you press the bar straight overhead (figure 4.30b). You have to lean slightly back and move your head back to avoid hitting your chin on the way up. Once the bar is straight overhead, adjust your posture so that you are standing tall with everything in alignment. Once at the top, take a deep breath in, hold strong for a moment, and lower the bar. Press it straight back up again and release your breath just enough to take more in.

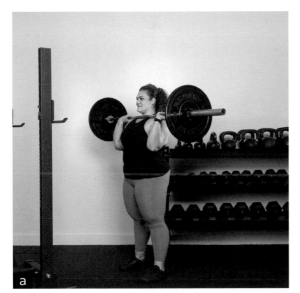 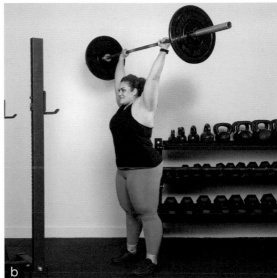

Figure 4.30 Barbell overhead press: *(a)* start position; *(b)* top position.

Tips and Tricks

Barbell overhead press is the fourth of the powerlifting movements. Although most competitions include squat, bench, and deadlift, some competitions include squat, press, and deadlift.

Shoulder Accessory Exercises

The next two movements are shoulder accessory exercises. The muscles used in these exercises are used in other exercises in this book. Isolated exercises for these small muscles are beneficial. My clients like to joke that when I take out the light weight, they get nervous. For the front raise and lateral raise, you aren't lifting much weight. Do a higher repetition range using lighter weight, no matter how strong you are.

Lateral Raise

Stand tall with a dumbbell in each hand, palms facing your thighs, arms at your sides (figure 4.31*a*). With straight arms (slight bend in the elbows is okay), raise your arms to shoulder height (figure 4.31*b*). Slowly lower arms back to start position and repeat.

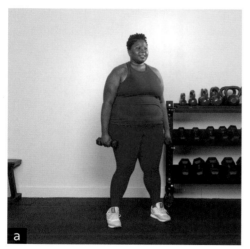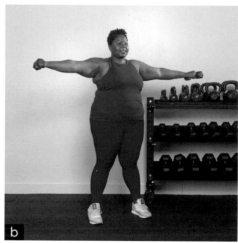

Figure 4.31   Lateral raise: *(a)* start position; *(b)* top position.

Muscles

Primary: Middle deltoid, upper trapezius, serratus anterior

Movement Focus

Focus on keeping your core tight and using only your arms to lift the weight. It's easy to try to cheat to lift the weights up to your sides. You may find that you try to use momentum. Pick a weight that allows you to lift with control. People who perform a lateral raise without control may start to feel tightness in their necks. The upper trapezius is working during a lateral raise, but if you focus on your shoulders and relax, you won't have pain in the neck.

Cues

- Keep your core tight.
- Straighten your arms.
- Relax your neck.

Front Raise

Stand tall with a dumbbell in each hand, arms on the outside of your thighs, palms facing your thighs (figure 4.32a). With straight arms, bring the weight straight up to shoulder height (figure 4.32b). Slowly bring the weight back down and repeat.

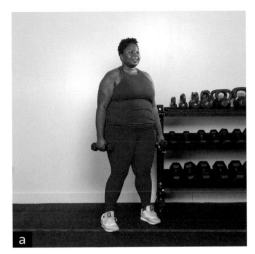 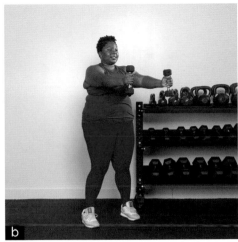

Figure 4.32   Front raise: (a) start position; (b) top position.

Muscles

Primary: Anterior deltoid

Secondary: Pectoralis, middle deltoid, trapezius

Movement Focus

Hold your core strong. Try not to use momentum to swing the weight up. This movement is usually done with a light weight so you can control the weight and use strength.

Cues

- Keep your core strong.
- Straighten your arms.

CONCLUSION

If you ask most people, they would say that women aren't as strong as men (insert sigh emoji). We have the ability to be as strong as we want to be, but it can be a lot harder to build upper-body strength than it is to build our lower bodies. It's equally important, though, so don't get discouraged. Be patient, get in those repetitions, and keep working at it. The biggest piece of advice I can give you about upper-body strength—actually, strength in general—is that the whole body works together. So, create tension: Use those legs and use that core, even when doing upper-body exercises. Using your whole body as one helps you get stronger and hit those goals, like completing those push-ups and pull-ups. In the next chapter we will go over core exercises, and then we will put it all together.

ANTI-ROTATION, LOADED CARRY, AND ROTATION

Core is life, but what does the term *core* really mean? Your core is the part of your body that stabilizes your spine, the part of your body that gets everything else working together. Many people think the core is only the abs. Yes, your abs are part of your core, but so is your butt, your chest, and your back. The core runs from your hips all the way to your shoulders; everything else is just an extremity.

The middle section of your body is very important (figure 5.1). Think about what lives underneath your abs: all of your vital organs and your spine. Like I said, core is life. The purpose of a strong core isn't a six-pack; we need to have a strong core to protect life.

Without the core, you wouldn't be able to squat, do push-ups, or deadlift. Some of the strongest people in the world have big bellies. Can you picture a world's strongest competitor, or a gymnast, or a CrossFit athlete? What's the one thing they all have in common? Wide, strong stomachs and wide backs. When I say big belly, I mean a rock-solid middle. I like to talk about the core as a brick wall. You may remember from bracing for your squat in chapter 3 that I spoke about breathing into your belly. This is like creating the brick wall, and it may be hard to find this feeling at first.

I want you to try something for me. Sit in a chair and think about pushing to use the bathroom. I know that sounds crazy, but in order to push, you have now created tension in your core and therefore are pressing into the brick wall! The other way I have taught clients to brace is by pretending to punch them in the stomach when they don't expect it. Let me be clear: I've never punched a client in the stomach. But if you think it's going to happen, it causes an automatic reaction of bracing your core. That bracing is important as the starting point of the core exercises you learn in this chapter.

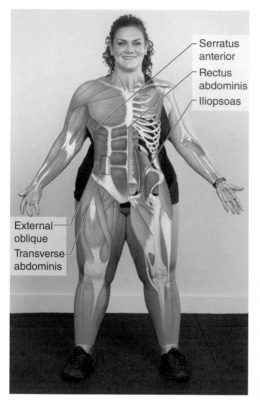
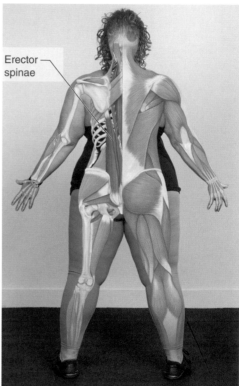

Figure 5.1   Muscles of the core.

ANTI-ROTATION

One of the main ways that we work core strength is through anti-rotation. Anti-rotation means just that: working to prevent rotation and to create stability of the spine. Different anti-rotation exercises each have a specific purpose.

Plank

Planking is the simplest form of core exercise there is. You don't have to do anything; you stay completely still and get stronger by doing so. But why are planks so hard? Any form of isometric hold, which means any exercise you do when you hold the position, is hard. Your muscles start to burn out and fatigue. A plank, specifically, is hard because you are holding your whole body up with your arms and feet, so everything in the middle has to be working together in order for your body to stay up.

We spoke briefly about plank position when we discussed push-ups. Remember my cue to be light as a feather, stiff as a board? Keep that in mind as I walk you through the instructions for how to perform a perfect plank.

Muscles

Primary: Rectus abdominis

Secondary: Obliques, iliopsoas, tensor fasciae latae, quadriceps, sartorius, pectoralis, serratus anterior, glutes, erector spinae

Instructions

Place your palms on the floor, stacking your wrists under the shoulders, and walk your feet back behind you so you're on your toes. Keep your abdomen strong with the belly button pulling up to the ceiling. Squeeze your butt and your legs and press the balls of the feet into the floor. Keep your head in line with your spine, looking at the floor just a little bit in front of you (figure 5.2). In order to do any version of a plank properly, your whole body must work together. You can hold your abdomen strong, but if you don't use your legs and squeeze your butt, you won't be in the best plank position possible.

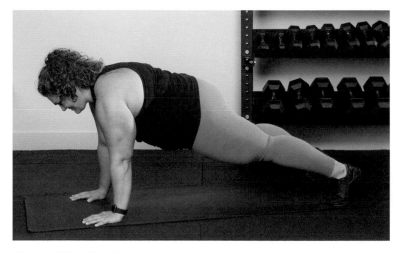

Figure 5.2 Plank position.

Movement Focus

Learning to plank properly may seem easy, but the body wants to do things to cheat, to make it feel easier. The biggest issue we see in planks is the same one we see in push-ups: the abdomen falling and the lower back arching. It may seem wrong, but you actually want to tuck your hips in, so squeeze your butt and pull your belly button up to the ceiling to create a safer position for your spine as well as a stronger position for your plank.

The other issue we see is placement of the hands. Your wrists and palms should be directly under your shoulders, but this can be really hard. Not everyone can immediately hold all their body weight on their wrists. Some people place their arms a little farther in front of them, and that's okay. Learning to hold yourself up in a safe position trumps being in the precisely correct position. As you get more comfortable on your wrists, you can slowly move them under the shoulders.

Cues

- Squeeze your butt.
- Pull your belly button up toward the ceiling.
- Press through the floor with your hands.

Variations

Hands Elevated Prone Plank

Use a box, a weight bench, or even a chair to elevate your plank (figure 5.3). This is a great way to take some of your body weight out of the equation and work on getting stronger in a plank position. When elevating themselves, people sometimes push their weight into the legs. Be sure to find proper alignment, keeping weight in your arms as well.

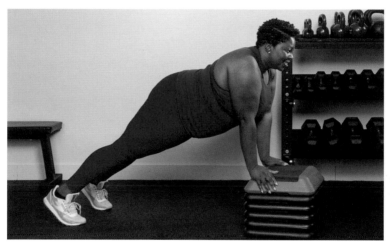

Figure 5.3   Hands elevated prone plank.

Kneeling Plank

If you are ready to try plank from the ground but have a hard time staying in the position for a long time, try the kneeling plank. Start from a full plank position and then drop your knees to the ground (figure 5.4). Check in with your body to make sure your hips are down and that you aren't in an all-fours position. Check that you are still squeezing your butt.

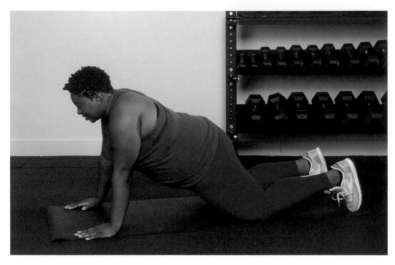

Figure 5.4   Kneeling plank.

Forearm Plank

Besides moving your palms a little farther out in a full plank to alleviate some of the pressure on the wrists, you can also work your plank position on your forearms. With your forearms on the ground, palms facing the ground and your shoulders and elbows aligned, the rest of your body is in the same position as your plank (figure 5.5).

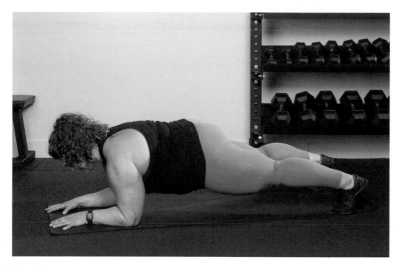

Figure 5.5   Forearm plank.

Kneeling Forearm Plank

Start on your forearms and the balls of your feet then drop your knees to the floor (figure 5.6). Check that you are still squeezing your butt and that your hips aren't too high in the air. Kneeling forearm plank is great if a full plank is too much for your core and lower back. You can still gain the strength benefits of a plank by shortening your position and therefore making it more doable.

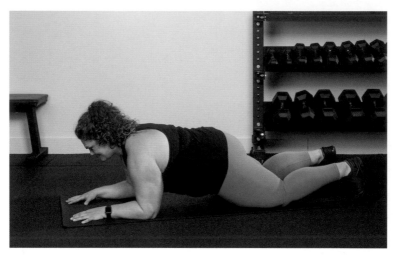

Figure 5.6   Kneeling forearm plank.

Forearm Side Plank

Lie on your side and place your forearm on the ground with your elbow underneath your shoulder. With your forearm and bottom foot touching the floor, your body should be in alignment as well as your elbow directly below your shoulder. Check that your hip isn't dipping to the ground and that your shoulder isn't riding up to your ear. Press your forearm and foot into the floor and press your body away from it to find a strong position (figure 5.7).

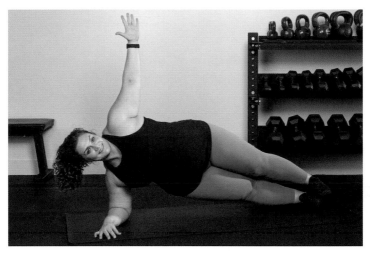

Figure 5.7   Forearm side plank.

Kneeling Side Plank

Lie on your side. Place your forearm on the ground with your elbow underneath your shoulder. Have your body aligned with your knees bent to about 90 degrees behind your body. Lift your hip off the ground. When you are up in your side plank, check that you're pressing through the floor with your forearm and bottom leg (figure 5.8).

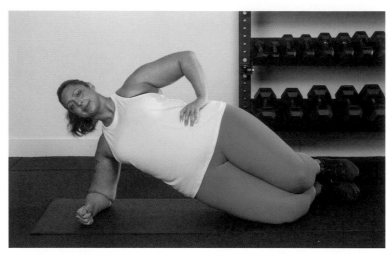

Figure 5.8   Kneeling side plank.

Pallof Press

Plank can be a hard exercise for people, especially in the beginning. So why not work on the core from a standing position? The core is tricky, and when not strong enough, people can feel lower-back pain. Standing anti-rotation exercises are a great way to get stronger without being on the floor, and they also don't put the lower back in a compromising position. The Pallof press is a great anti-rotation exercise with a couple of variations.

Muscles

Primary: Obliques, transverse abdominis, scapular stabilizers, glutes, rectus abdominis

Instructions

Using a cable machine or a resistance band, stand with your side next to its attachment point. The cable or resistance band should be at about your midsection. Place your hands around the handle with fingers interlaced, and step out away from the attachment point so that there is resistance (figure 5.9a). Stand with your feet about hip-width apart, slightly bend your knees, squeeze your butt, brace your core, and lift your chest. Press the band or cable straight out in front of you (figure 5.9b), hold at the end point for at least two counts, and slowly bring it back in toward your body. The resistance is coming from the side, and it's your job when pressing out not to let it pull you to that side.

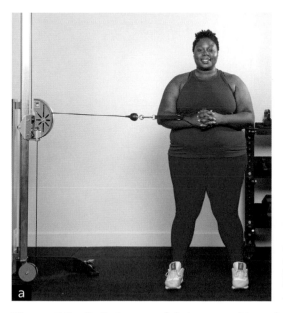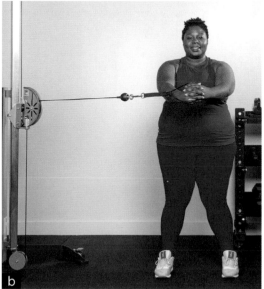

Figure 5.9 Pallof press: (a) start position; (b) end position (arms straight).

Movement Focus

We control the weight; the weight doesn't control us. In a Pallof press, if you are being pulled in the direction of the cable, it's probably a little too heavy or you aren't focused on keeping control of the weight. Remember it might feel lighter when you are closer to your body, but when you have pressed that weight away from you and your arms are out straight, it feels much heavier and harder. That is where it matters most. Any of the anti-rotation movements can in theory sound or look easy, but it's what you put into the move that matters most. Are you focused on holding strong, concentrating on a good core position? Are you able to breathe, even at the hardest point? Remember to breathe, remember to check in that your shoulders are down and away from your ears. Each time you press the weight out, you risk hiking your shoulders up to your ears. Remember that while this is a core exercise, your back and shoulders are part of your core.

Cues

- Lock your body in place.
- Bring your shoulders down.
- Brace your abdominal muscles.

Variations

Half Kneeling Pallof Press

The arm movement is the same, but the legs are in the kneeling position (figure 5.10). With both knees on the ground, you use your butt and core even more than when you perform this exercise from a standing position.

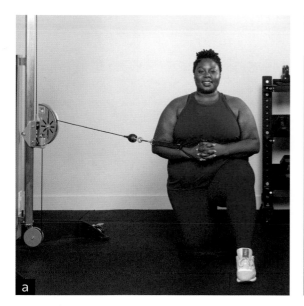 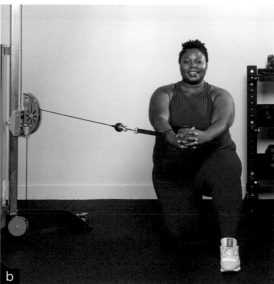

Figure 5.10 Half kneeling Pallof press: *(a)* start position; *(b)* end position (arms straight).

Woodchop

Stand tall with the knees slightly bent, abdomen strong, and hips locked in place (figure 5.11a). The cable is set in a high position, just above the head. Using straight arms, pull the cable across the body (figure 5.11b) and slowly bring it back to the beginning. Expect some upper-body (thoracic) rotation, but the legs, hips, and core are locked in place.

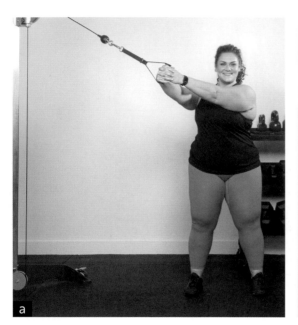 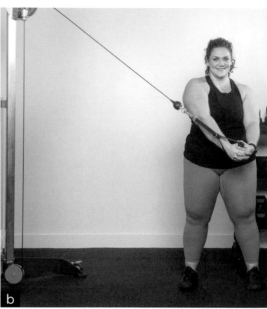

Figure 5.11   Woodchop: *(a)* start position; *(b)* end position (arms across body).

Half Kneeling Woodchop

Assume a half kneeling position with the knee closest to the cable or band on the ground and the outside leg bent to 90 degrees with the foot on the floor (figure 5.12a). The cable is set above shoulder height. Pull the cable to just above the outside leg (figure 5.12b) and slowly return it back to the beginning. Make sure not to lean into the outside leg too much; put even weight into the ground and lock your lower half into place on the pull and the return.

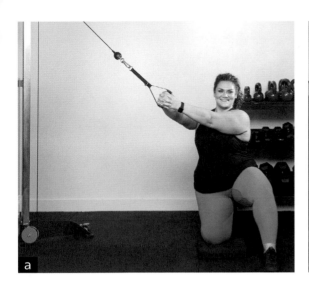 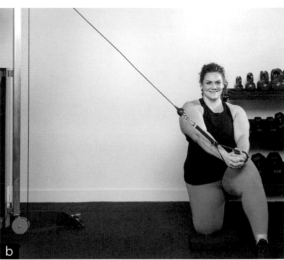

Figure 5.12 Half kneeling woodchop: *(a)* start position; *(b)* end position.

Split Stance Woodchop

Set the cable to just above shoulder height while you are standing next to it. The split stance woodchop is similar to the half kneeling woodchop except this time your back knee won't rest on the ground. Hold yourself in a split squat position (figure 5.13a) and pull the weight toward the outside leg (figure 5.13b). This takes a lot of balance and coordination; holding your body in a split squat is hard enough and adding being pulled by the weight is a whole new ball game. Keep the hips from moving as the upper body pulls the weight across your body.

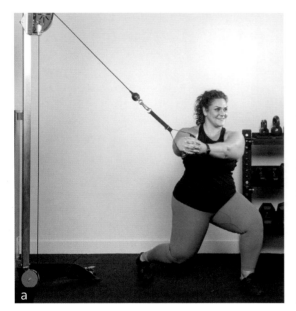 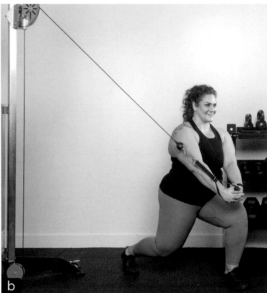

Figure 5.13 Split stance woodchop: *(a)* start position; *(b)* end position.

LOADED CARRY

Loaded carries are a form of anti-rotation movements, like the exercises in the previous section. However, when walking or in gait, you automatically rotate the hips. Think about walking home while carrying heavy bags; that is a loaded carry. Now picture that while you are walking, the bags are swinging all over the place, making it much harder to carry your bags home. During loaded carries, we absolutely have natural movement of the body while creating anti-rotation of the core to control the equipment. Loaded carries can be done in different ways, but generally speaking, you are walking with heavy weight and focusing on your core.

Farmer's Carry

Farmer's carries are probably one of the simplest yet most efficient ways to get stronger. Your core, legs, and upper body—and just about every muscle in your body—are forced to work when doing any variation of a farmer's carry.

Farmer's carries are simply picking up some weight and carrying it from one place to another. I like to joke with my clients that if you need to get the six-packs to the party, you have to carry them there. It's actually more like when you go to the grocery store and have two heavy bags to get home. We do farmer's carries all the time in our daily activities. Now if we put a little focus into what we are doing and add a certain distance, it becomes an exercise. It can be easy to bend over, pick up a weight, and walk, but when we do any form of movement, we should be focused on what we are doing. In this case, when picking up the weight, you are doing a suitcase deadlift (page 52).

Muscles

All muscles (the whole body is working)

Instructions

To perform the suitcase deadlift to get into position for the farmer's carry, hinge from your hips, keep your abdomen braced, and grab a weight in each hand (figure 5.14a). Use kettlebells, dumbbells, or specific farmer's carry bars. Stand tall, open your chest, and pull your shoulders away from your ears (figure 5.14b). Minimize rotation of the hips. Take several steps and bend the knees to set the weight back down on the ground.

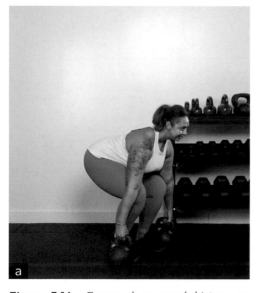 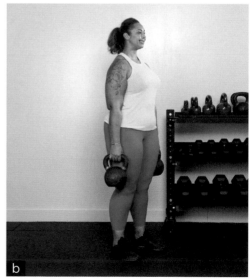

Figure 5.14 Farmer's carry: *(a)* hinge to pick up the weight; *(b)* stand.

Movement Focus

What tends to happen when walking with weight is that the chest wants to fall because the weight pulls us down. It's our job to train that core strength and stay tall. Use your body; think about the core, the back, and the chest all staying strong and working together. When you are walking with weights, momentum tends to take over. The weights may start to swing; one of your jobs while doing a farmer's carry is to prevent the weights from moving around. Remember that a farmer's carry is an anti-rotation exercise. When you walk, there is rotation of the hips. This is natural and should happen, but, ideally, we are working to keep the core still and strong and not let the weights determine what our bodies do.

Cues

- Walk slowly with control.
- Keep your chest tall.
- Prevent the weight from swinging.

Variations

Single-Arm Farmer's Carry

Use the suitcase deadlift technique to pick up a weight in one hand only (figure 5.15). The challenge with this exercise is that the weight wants to pull you down to the side you are holding it on. To offset this, you must focus on your core and pretend as if you have weight evenly distributed in both arms. If you find that one side is much harder than the other, this may be a great exercise to do more repetitions or sets on that side.

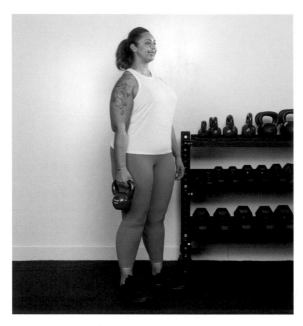

Figure 5.15   Single-arm farmer's carry standing position.

Front Rack Farmer's Carry

In a front rack farmer's carry, you can use dumbbells or kettlebells (figure 5.16). Either way, you have to get the weight up to your chest. With dumbbells, hold the weights just above the shoulders with your chest high. With kettlebells, the weights rest on the outside of each wrist, with your knuckles touching. No matter what you use, the weight should be sitting right above your chest. You need to work hard to keep it up. The weight wants to pull you down. While a front rack farmer's carry is very much a core exercise, it is without a doubt also a back exercise. You should feel your midback working to hold a strong posture. It is normal to have a slight lean in your lower back, but if it gets excessive, you should probably reduce the amount of weight you're holding.

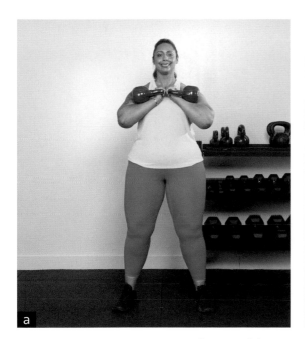
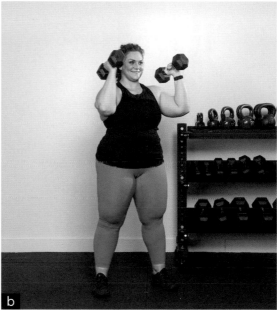

Figure 5.16 Front rack farmer's carry: (a) kettlebell front rack farmer's carry standing position; (b) dumbbell front rack farmer's carry standing position.

> ### *Tips and Tricks*
> Don't let your forearms rest on your chest. It's okay if they touch, but rest means you are no longer using your strength to hold up the weight.

Overhead Farmer's Carry

Use your suitcase deadlift technique (page 52) to pick up a weight in each hand. Using your overhead shoulder press technique (page 97), press the weights straight overhead (figure 5.17). With arms in line with the ears, start walking. Be sure to press the weight away from you while maintaining tension in your core and keeping your shoulders down and away from your ears. If you have a hard time with shoulder press and overhead mobility, do not perform this exercise until you can do it without any pain.

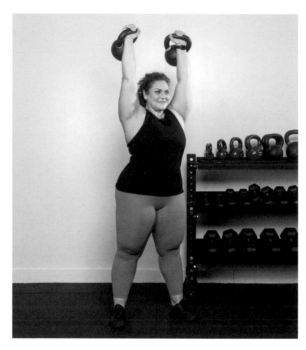

Figure 5.17   Overhead farmer's carry standing position.

ROTATION

The body naturally rotates as we walk, grab something, or pull a door open. We rotate through the hips and spine. These movements happen naturally, but we can make them stronger. Here are some rotational strength movements. Over time they can also be done with speed and power.

Cable Rotation

Band and cable rotation exercises are really fun. They can be done slowly and controlled, which I recommend that you master first before you try doing them fast and with a lot of power. Anti-rotation exercises are super important for getting strong, learning how to brace the core, and protecting the spine. But in life, we move and rotate, and so we want to work our bodies in more realistic ways, as well. This is where rotation exercises come in. With the band or cable rotation exercises in this section, we involve the hips to make the movements more functional.

Muscles

Primary: Rectus abdominis, obliques, transverse abdominis, glutes
Secondary: Scapular stabilizers

Instructions

Stand with one side next to the band or cable at about midstomach height. Grab the handle with fingers interlaced. Step out away from the attachment point so that there is resistance. Straighten your arms, with your hands close to the attachment point (figure 5.18a). As you bring the weight across your body, rotate your hips to face away from the machine or band (figure 5.18b). Hold the end position for at least one second and then, with straight arms, slowly rotate back to the start position.

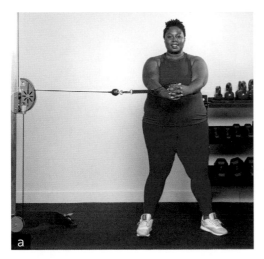 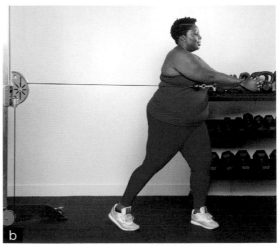

Figure 5.18   Cable rotation: *(a)* start position; *(b)* end position (arms away from anchor).

Movement Focus

Cable rotations help you work on powerful movements, but what can tend to happen is that you rotate through the wrong parts of your body. Sometimes people rotate through the lower back, but the lower back has only about 5 to 15 degrees of rotation. The focus needs to come from the hips and legs. As you follow through the rotation, be sure that you are bringing your hips with you so that they face away from the attachment point of the cable or band.

Cues

- Rotate through your hips.
- Straighten your arms.
- Brace your abdominal muscles.

Variations

Half Kneeling Rotation

In a half kneeling position, with the knee closest to the cable or band (at midabdomen height) on the ground and the outside leg bent to 90 degrees with foot on the floor (figure 5.19a), pull the cable to just past the outside leg (figure 5.19b) and slowly return to the beginning. Make sure not to lean into the outside leg too much; put even weight into the ground. This is similar to the woodchop (page 118), but let your hips open to the machine and close when pulling the cable or band over the knee.

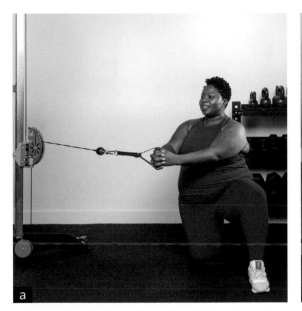
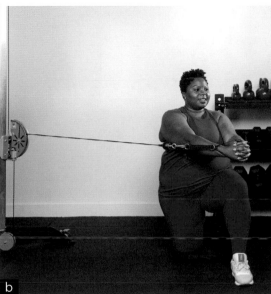

Figure 5.19   Half kneeling rotation: *(a)* start position; *(b)* end position.

Split Stance Rotation

Standing next to the cable machine with the side of your body facing the machine, place the cable at midabdomen height. Step out while holding the cable with both hands wrapped around the handle. Step away from the cable machine. Step the leg closest to the machine back and bend the back knee so that you are now in a split squat position (page 60). Once in a split squat (figure 5.20a), pull the weight toward the outside leg (figure 5.20b). This is like the split stance woodchop (page 120), but this time you let your hips open to the machine and rotate closed when you pull toward the knee.

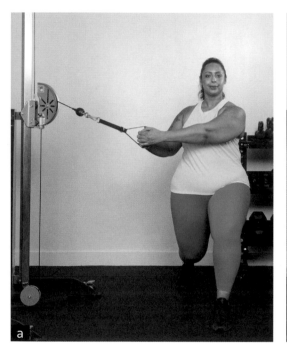 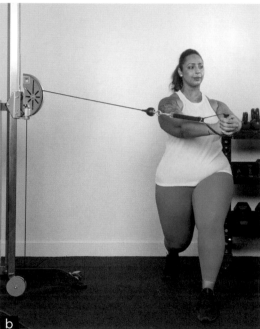

Figure 5.20   Split stance rotation: (a) start position; (b) end position.

CONCLUSION

The exercise library is huge. I'm not even sure how many exercises there actually are. Anything can be an exercise. Any movement done with purpose can be considered an exercise. The last three chapters have covered basic strength movements—rigid movement, purposeful movement. Remember to take your time and adjust so that you feel comfortable with what you are doing—but not too comfortable because exercise and strength training are supposed to be hard. The body works as a whole, not piece by piece. Create tension in your body, remember to breathe, and focus on what you are doing. We all have unique bodies that move differently, so adjust as necessary. The next few chapters take the movements we learned and put them together to create a program that helps you reach your goals.

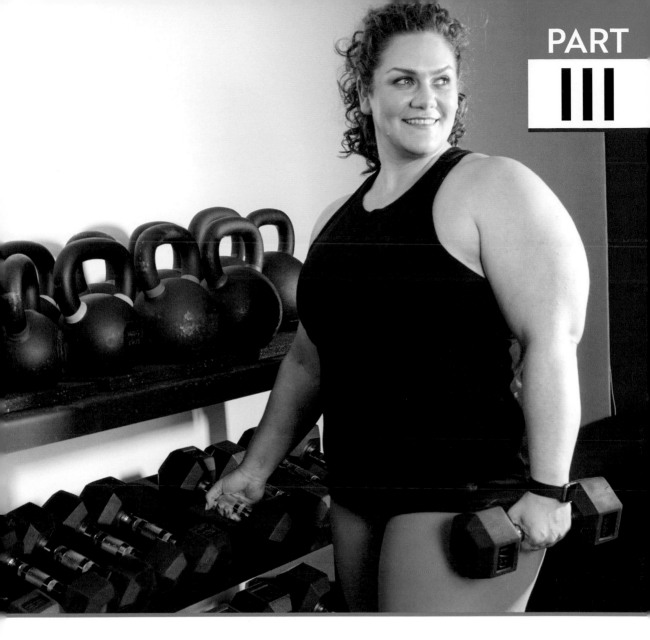

Make a Plan

CHAPTER

CREATE YOUR WORKOUT

Now that you have gone through chapters 3, 4, and 5 and you understand the movements to use to get stronger, let's put a workout together. You probably don't want to walk into a gym without knowing what to do. We need to know what movements to do, how to do them, and when to do them. There are different ways we can go about this. There isn't a right or a wrong way to train. The goal is to figure out what works for you and what is efficient and smart training.

A lot of fitness experts out there talk about exercise versus training. What's the difference? Exercise, to me, is just moving for the sake of movement, not having a plan, doing whatever you want within the realm of fitness. Training is all about the body, the mind, and working toward something. I clearly believe in training, in setting goals, committing to them, and sticking to a plan. It works for me and I like to be compliant with a plan. However, I don't actually believe there is anything wrong with exercise. I've said it before and I'll say it again, even if people don't agree with me. I would rather you do something than nothing. But it can't hurt to try sticking to a plan, so let's talk about the different ways to create a training plan so you can get started.

GOAL SETTING

In chapter 2, we talked about why and how to set a goal. Let's take your goal and talk about how it determines what kind of workout plan you take on. If I want to run a marathon, I shouldn't be swimming every day. If I want to be able to do push-ups, I'm going to need to do push-ups. If you want to get stronger, you need to lift. If you want to move faster, you need to lift and then work on power. The goal that you pick helps determine the direction in which your plan takes you. Simply put, if you want to work on an upper-body strength goal, your program needs to lean heavily toward upper-body strength. If you are looking to increase your back squat or deadlift, your program is going to have to lean heavily toward those movements and the lower body. As a reminder, your body and muscles don't work independently from each other. This means that even with wanting to improve push-ups or pull-ups or the upper body in general, I still need to work on the lower body and core. It's never a good idea to only do one thing. It is, however, okay to lean more heavily toward something.

Repetition and practice are always necessary to get better at something; exercise and strength are no different. Our bodies adapt over time. We become more comfortable with movements and weights. Let's say that you are a beginner who wants to get stronger with a focus on being able to do 10 full push-ups, and you have the availability to work out three times a week. You want a plan that incorporates three full-body strength days. In chapter 7, there are a few examples of training plans that could work for you, but if you have a goal of doing push-ups, you need to be doing push-ups. As a beginner, pick variations that work for you. For example, a hands elevated push-up helps you focus on your range of motion and form. After a few weeks of patterning the movement and increasing your repetitions, you realize it's time to take the incline down, and you continue this pattern until you are doing push-ups on the floor. Maybe one day a week you are doing hands elevated push-ups, and another day during the week you are working on your planks. Remember a push-up is a plank with motion, so working on your plank helps you get to your goal. All movements can relate to one another. Figuring out what feels weak for you helps determine what movements you put in your program to help hit your goals. If I go to perform a push-up and my stomach is drooping, I should be working on holding my core strong. If I go to do a push-up and my chest and triceps give out, maybe I need to add more chest exercises. When I first started powerlifting and I was doing more squats and bench presses, my push-ups by default got so much stronger. I was generally getting stronger, but I was also figuring out how to create more tension in my body while doing push-ups.

If you've created a plan based on your goals, stuck to it for at least four weeks, and aren't seeing any improvement, change it up. Try something different. Maybe for you the hands elevated push-up wasn't the way to go and negative push-ups are a better idea. But, generally speaking, if you stick to something and keep practicing and get those repetitions in, you're going to get stronger. Now that you have some idea of how to take your goal and implement it, let's work on the steps of creating your workout plan.

WARM UP

Let's start with warming up as part of each workout. It is probably one of the most important things you can do because you need to prime the body. Think of your body as a rubber band; if it's been sitting in a cold car for a long time and you pull it, what happens? The rubber band rips. In the body, if our muscles, tendons, ligaments, and fascia are cold and we don't work our way into the workout, we can end up with an injury.

The warm-up looks different for each training program, but no matter what kind of warm-up you do, there should always be one. It could be something simple, such as a five-minute treadmill walk, a dynamic mobility warm-up, or even barbell drills. Which warm-up is used depends on the person, her body, and her program. If you are a morning workout person, you were recently sleeping all night long and you aren't truly awake yet, so your body needs to be woken up before it can work. If you are an after-work person, you were probably sitting all day and now you are stiff and tired. Either way, you need to warm up. Especially if you are new to strength training, I highly recommend taking the time to warm up, even if it means less time for the actual workout. The goal is longevity, to be able to keep training and lifting for a long time. In order to do that, you want to prevent injury, and one of the ways to do that is by prepping the body for the workout.

Warm-up movements are exercises. It takes time to get better and more comfortable with these exercises, like any part of your workout. You have options for warming up, but each movement should have a purpose. For that reason, warming up is sometimes called movement prep. In strength training, you shouldn't start squatting with 400 pounds on your back. You want to prep the body for what is to come. For example, if the muscles in my chest are tight, getting under the bar for a back squat could be really difficult. But if I take the time to warm up my shoulders and chest, it is easier to get myself under the bar.

There is no exact prescription for warm-ups and no specific number of reps and sets you should do. The idea is to get your body warm, your blood flowing, and your body loose, all with intention. It's a time to focus on your breath, movement patterns, and mindfulness. I could tell you to do 5 to 10 repetitions of any of the movements that follow, but if you feel you need more or fewer, then you should go with that gut feeling for what your body needs. Here are some of my favorite warm-up movements. This group of exercises hits all different parts of the body and includes variations so you can adjust the exercises to suit your body.

Cat–Cow

Purpose

Spinal mobility and breath work

Instructions

Begin on all fours. Slowly round your back by tucking your tailbone and hips and rounding your spine toward the ceiling (cat; figure 6.1a). Be sure to tuck your chin into your chest and push away from the ground with your hands and knees. Your back should be as round as possible. To move into cow (figure 6.1b), slowly reverse the motion of your tailbone and hips and let your belly release toward the floor as you stretch through the front of your body. Be sure to pull your shoulder blades away from your ears. When in cow position, check that you feel your lats engaged. I like to teach cat and cow not only for spinal mobility but also as a deadlift warm-up. When you move into cow and you pull your shoulders away from your ears, you use your back muscles to do it. This is exactly what you do when you engage the back and shoulders for your deadlift setup. Move slowly through this movement, focusing on your spine, hips, and shoulder blades.

Cat–cow is also a great opportunity to focus on your breath. When rounding your spine to the ceiling, you are closing your diaphragm, so this is where the exhale happens; push as far as you can in both body and breath. As you slowly transition to cow, your diaphragm opens, and you should inhale and take in as much air as possible through your belly.

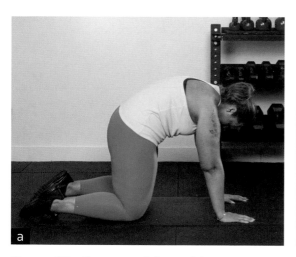
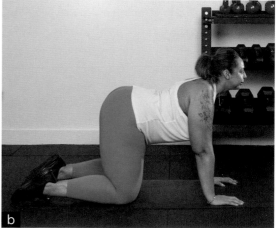

Figure 6.1   Cat–cow: (a) cat; (b) cow.

Seated Cat–Cow

Purpose

Spinal mobility and breath work

Instructions

Sit tall with your feet planted on the ground. As you begin a long exhale, slowly let your back round toward the back of the chair while your hips tuck under and your shoulders round into your chest (cat; figure 6.2a). With your next inhale, slowly sit up tall, pushing your hips toward the back of the chair and letting your chest come forward as far as it can (cow; figure 6.2b). Repeat the process slowly and with intention.

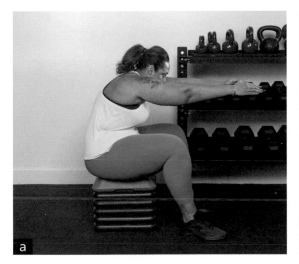 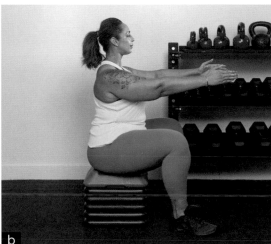

Figure 6.2   Seated cat–cow: *(a)* cat; *(b)* cow.

Bird Dog

Purpose

Build core strength, stability, and coordination

Instructions

Begin on all fours. Extend one arm long in line with your ears as you extend the opposite leg straight out behind you (figure 6.3). Continue to press through the floor with the hand and knee still on the floor and hold your abdomen strong; don't let your lower back and abdomen sag. Try to get your lifted leg in line with the body; a little higher is okay, but you don't want to overextend the hips and arch the lower back. You can alternate sides or stick to one side at a time. Remember to breathe: Inhale while you extend your arms and legs and exhale when you return to the middle. This is one of my favorite warm-ups and a great way to work on spinal stability while warming up your extremities.

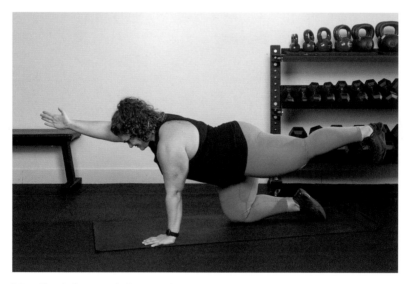

Figure 6.3 Bird dog with leg and arm extended.

Spider Lunge

Purpose

Stretch the hips and hamstrings

Instructions

From a plank position (figure 6.4*a*), step one foot up as close to the outside of your hand as possible. Aim for full extension in the hips (let the hips sink toward the floor while keeping your back leg straight) and a long spine (lift the chest and keep the neck in line with the spine; figure 6.4*b*). Take a deep breath, bring your foot back to plank position, and switch sides. You can also perform this stretch from a plank position on a box or bench (figure 6.4*c*).

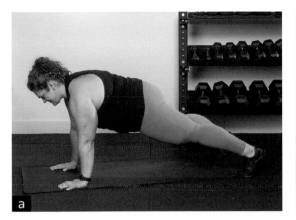
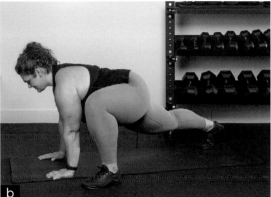
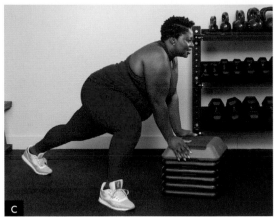

Figure 6.4 Spider lunge: *(a)* plank; *(b)* spider lunge on the floor; *(c)* spider lunge on a box or bench.

Quadruped Thoracic Rotation

Purpose

Midback and upper-back mobility, breath work

Instructions

Begin on all fours. Place one hand behind your head (figure 6.5a). Rotate to lift your elbow and open your chest to the sky (figure 6.5b). This is a great place to work on breath as well: Exhale as you rotate toward the sky and inhale as you return to the start position. Switch sides.

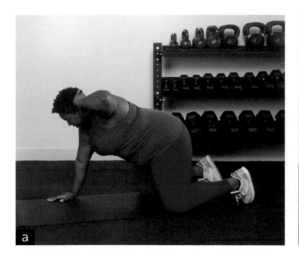 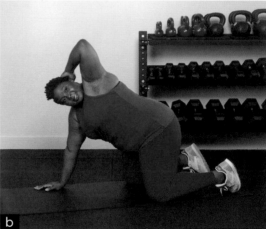

Figure 6.5   Quadruped thoracic rotation: *(a)* start position; *(b)* rotated position.

Supine T-Spine Opener

Purpose

Midback and upper-back mobility, breath work

Instructions

Lie on your side with the knees bent 90 degrees and stacked on one another, arms stretched out in front of you (figure 6.6a). You may want to place a block, pillow, or foam roller under your head. Keep your bottom arm flat on the floor, and now slowly lift your top arm in an arc over your body as you reach for the ground on the opposite side, letting your chest open (figure 6.6b). Exhale while opening, and inhale while closing. Switch sides.

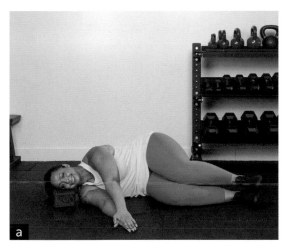 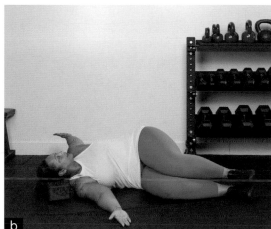

Figure 6.6 Supine T-spine opener: *(a)* start position; *(b)* open.

Bridge

Purpose

Activate and strengthen the glutes

Instructions

Lie on your back with your knees bent and feet flat on the floor, arms beside you with the palms on the ground (figure 6.7a). Squeeze your glutes and push your lower back into the floor. Keep squeezing as you push down through your feet and press your hips up toward the ceiling (figure 6.7b). Be sure not to overextend and push up with your lower back; instead, focus on extending through your hips. Lower your hips back to the floor and repeat. If your hamstrings start to cramp, you likely need to step your feet a bit farther from your body. If you don't feel your glutes, you are likely using your lower back in your extension.

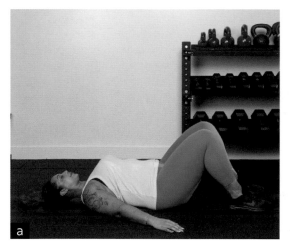 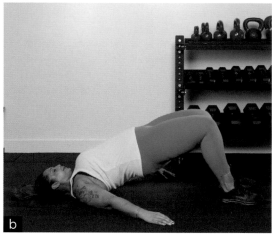

Figure 6.7 Bridge: *(a)* start position; *(b)* press hips up.

Reverse Crunch

Purpose

Activate and strengthen the core

Instructions

Lie on your back with your knees bent and feet in the air so that your legs make approximately a 90-degree angle (figure 6.8a). Press your lower back into the floor and slowly lower your heels to tap the ground, keeping your knees bent the whole time (figure 6.8b). As you lower your heels toward the floor, keep pressing your whole back into the ground to keep your lower back and shoulders from coming off the floor. As an alternative, you can lower one leg at a time and alternate legs.

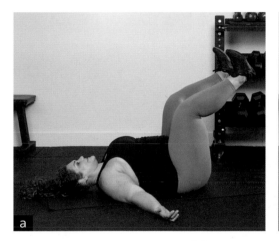 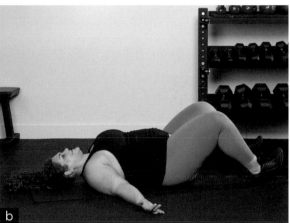

Figure 6.8 Reverse crunch: *(a)* start position; *(b)* lower heels.

Shoulder Dislocates

Purpose

Shoulder mobility

Instructions

Each version of a shoulder dislocates is intended to help you work on shoulder mobility and range of motion. Here is an easy one to start with. Use a PVC pipe, Swiffer stick, broomstick, or another long, thin, lightweight object. Hold the stick in front of your hips with a wide grip and straight arms, and slowly raise it all the way over your head (figure 6.9a). Keep going past your head as far as you are comfortable, bringing your arms behind you (figure 6.9b). Be sure to go slowly and move with control; you don't want to injure your shoulder. Reverse the motion to come back to the start position. Repeat a few times and try to slowly move your hands closer and closer together. The narrower the grip, the greater the stretch. As your grip narrows, it is okay to bend your elbows and pull the bar down behind your head (figure 6.9c). This helps you get more comfortable with being in a back squat position.

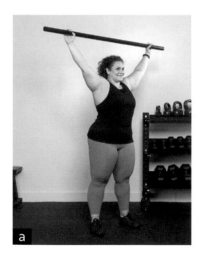 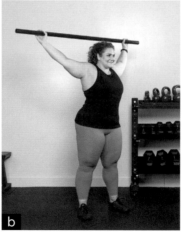 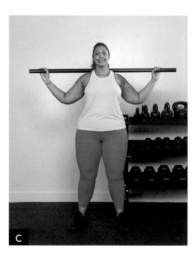

Figure 6.9 Shoulder dislocates: (a) stick above head; (b) stick behind; (c) stick behind with elbows bent.

THE WORKOUT

When putting together your workout, think about which exercises feel the hardest or use the most energy. Generally, you should start a workout with exercises that use the bigger muscles and compound movements, such as squats or deadlifts, before moving to exercises that work the smaller muscles and single-joint movements, such as biceps curls. For example, my glutes are much bigger and stronger than my shoulders, so I would start my workout with a leg exercise versus a shoulder exercise. For the sake of this book, which is geared toward beginner strength, we are working with a full-body training program.

In a full-body training program, you use each part of your body in every workout in a week. We make sure that we aren't focused too much on one part of the body. In chapters 3, 4, and 5, all the movements are written in the order of most important to least important. They are written using the biggest muscle groups to smallest muscle groups within each category. When writing your program, you should do the same. Working our way from big muscle groups to small muscle groups is step one. The movements are also in our daily movement patterns: push, pull, hinge, squat, lunge, walk, and rotate. When we program, we want to make sure these movements are evenly distributed. The workouts in chapter 7 will be organized in this way.

Split Days

Many people use what is called a split-day training program. *Split days* simply means that you break up a full-body workout into separate workout days. You might divide the workout by lower body and upper body or even by different body parts. You have options. You could have a four-day-a-week training program with two lower-body days and two upper-body days. You could have a training program with a chest day, leg day, back day, and core day. These are examples, but no matter what kind of program you pick, order of movements is important. First perform compound movements, exercises that involve more than one body part. For example, on a leg day, I would start with a squat or a deadlift before moving to a lunge. The squat and deadlift use all the muscles in the body and multiple joints, and therefore are considered compound exercises. I could then move into the single-joint or less compound-heavy movements. If your goal is to get stronger and do so by lifting heavy weight, you don't want to tire out your body by starting with biceps curls. You want to start with pull-ups or back exercises. There are times that it makes sense to do things differently, but, as a general rule of thumb, start with the movements that use the most muscle groups or big muscle groups and then work toward the smaller muscle groups.

THREE STAGES OF LEARNING

In the same way we must allow time for our bodies to adapt to movements, our brains adjust, too, based on the way we learn new things. The three stages of learning are cognitive, associative, and autonomous.

During the cognitive phase, you take in information. You see the most gains here, but your workouts and memory for movements are the most inconsistent. In this stage, you try to put together all the pieces of the puzzle. You may be in this stage the longest.

During the associative phase, you take the information you have learned and use it. This is usually where most of your time is spent. Taking pieces of information and putting them into action helps you see small gains over time. Although you make adjustments during this stage, it still isn't perfect. You shouldn't expect perfection, but you will start to understand and learn how to fix movements or techniques to make them work best for you.

Finally, in the autonomous phase, after tons of practice and repetitions, the puzzle is complete. You find that a movement suddenly comes easily to you. This doesn't mean an exercise is easy. It means that you don't need to overthink how to do the exercise. This is where you want to be to progress the movement. It could take years to get to the autonomous phase. The interesting thing about the autonomous phase is that in strength training, you will likely be in the autonomous phase for only a short time. You will continue to add weight or progress your movement, so the autonomous phase is short lived.

The rate of progression is probably the biggest question when writing a strength training program. When can I progress? At what point do I automatically know how to perform an exercise? You know when your body and brain work together, not against each other. Progressing a movement is different than progressing weight, and I want to make that clear. You can progress a movement when you automatically know how to do it without doubt or hesitation. You can progress weight when it's appropriate, which is when your form stays intact and you can get through the allotted repetition range without struggle. Every time you master a weight or a movement, you make it a little bit harder by choosing a different variation, adding weight, changing tempo, or even changing rest periods.

REPETITIONS, SETS, REST, AND TEMPO

When you are new to any type of activity, you can go in blind and see results. You don't need much of a plan because your body reacts to any new stimulus. However, this won't last long. If your goal is to get stronger, it's time to make a plan. When programming strength training, there is a broad range in the definition of *strength*. Generally, programming for a powerlifting strength goal means doing 1 to 5 repetitions per set using a heavier weight, with long rest periods between sets. However, the exact numbers depend on your goal and fitness level. Strength can be gained by doing repetitions in the higher ranges. You hear and see different definitions of and opinions about strength. In the powerlifting world, strength training is defined as no more than 6 repetitions; however, if you are new to lifting, you are probably living in the range of 8 to 12 repetitions. Your body needs to acclimate to weight training and it would be unsafe to start with loads heavy enough that you could do only 6 repetitions or fewer. More senior lifters or stronger lifters are working their way to that one-repetition maximum (1RM). To reach that goal, they lift more weight for fewer repetitions over time. Their bodies and tissues are primed for heavier weights. Progressing too soon exposes you to injury. When patterning movement and slowly adding weight, your body needs to adjust so that injury does not occur. You shouldn't be able to do a lot of repetitions with a lot of weight. A newer lifter starts with more repetitions to ingrain patterns and slowly adds weight so that her body can adapt. Work your way up to lifting heavier weights. Take your time, follow the plan, and I promise you will get stronger.

Table 6.1 offers a look at the traditional suggested training volumes for different training goals. While I invite you to review these ranges, it is important to recognize that these estimates may not work for everyone. Also, remember you need to acclimate your bodies; don't do too much too soon. The two categories most relevant for this book are muscular hypertrophy and muscular strength, and my recommendations for hypertrophy-focused programs and max strength programs will follow, but I do feel it is important for you to understand different goals and how training changes to meet those goals.

Within the realm of strength training, there are two major categories where we want to live: hypertrophy and maximum (or max) strength. Hypertrophy simply means muscle growth, and since you probably picked up this book because you want to build muscle, the sample workouts you find here train primarily in the hypertrophy realm. A hypertrophy-focused program calls

Table 6.1 Training Volume Based on Goal

Training goal	Sets	Repetitions	Rest period	Intensity
General muscle fitness	1 or 2	15	30 to 90 sec	Varies
Muscular endurance	2 or 3	≥ 12	≤ 30 sec	60 to 70% 1RM
Muscular hypertrophy	3 to 6	6 to 12	30 to 90 sec	70 to 80% 1RM
Muscular strength	2 to 6	≤ 6	2 to 5 min	80 to 90% 1RM
Power: Single-effort events	3 to 5	1 or 2	2 to 5 min	> 90% 1RM
Power: Multiple-effort events	3 to 5	3 to 5	2 to 5 min	> 90% 1RM

1RM = One-repetition maximum

Data from T.R. Baechle and R.W. Earle, *Essentials of Strength Training and Conditioning,* 3rd ed. (Champaign, IL: Human Kinetics, 2008); W.L. Westcott, *Building Strength and Stamina,* 2nd ed. (Champaign, IL: Human Kinetics, 2003).

for 8 to 12 repetitions of each exercise per set, a total of 3 to 5 sets, and 1 to 2 minutes of rest between sets. In comparison, max strength means that you perform 1 to 6 repetitions per set, for 4 to 6 sets, and 2 to 5 minutes of rest between sets. These numbers vary depending on your specific needs and who writes the program, but you can see that there is a pretty big difference in the number of repetitions, sets, and minutes of rest. Let's look closer at why the numbers are different for these two types of strength training.

When you want to grow muscle in a hypertrophy stage, the more volume (repetitions) you do, the more your muscle grows. If you have never lifted before, this is the best place to start if your goal is to get stronger and build muscle mass. Over time, when you have built some muscle and are no longer a novice, you can transition to max strength.

Max strength training has a much smaller repetition range, because if you are lifting as much weight as possible, you simply shouldn't be able to do a lot of reps. Remember the goal is to lift as much as possible. Even so, there are very few people who train for strength and ONLY train in the numbers of max strength. For example, most programs use max strength numbers for the major lifts and use hypertrophy numbers for accessory lifts, like a biceps curl. When writing a program for strength, you probably have a mix of both hypertrophy and max strength training.

Another reason for using a range of repetitions, sets, and rest periods is to progress your workouts. To make progress, you can't let your body become acclimated. If you do the same repetitions and sets or even the same movements over and over again, you stop seeing progress because you're not challenging your body.

While you can do 8 to 12 repetitions in a hypertrophy-focused program, it would be smart to start closer to 12 repetitions with a weight that you can handle. The lower the number of repetitions you do, the more weight you should be lifting, and when you're starting out, you want to give your body time to adjust to the weights. If you try to lift weights that are heavier than your body is ready for, you may feel okay in the moment, but you risk feeling bad later or getting injured. Programming isn't just about writing down the exercises, repetitions, sets, and rest; it's about paying attention to your recovery and how you are responding to training. If after every workout you are unable to walk or lift your arms, you are doing too much. The goal isn't to be sore all the time. I suggest erring on the side of caution. I believe we are all capable, but I also believe that we should train smart. You have all the time in the world to add weight and sets. Start slowly, pay attention to how your body feels, and progress from there.

Adding weight isn't the only way to progress a program. Tempo is a fantastic way to progress a movement when working on strength. In an earlier chapter, we talked about creating tension in the body when doing your movements. When we add tempo to movements, we are increasing the time under tension (TUT). This results in more muscle fiber recruitment, which leads to muscle growth.

There is no rule for what tempo to use for an exercise. Start with something simple; let's use the squat as an example. As you perform your squat, count to three while you lower, pause for two seconds at the bottom, count to two as you come back up, and pause for two seconds at the top to breathe and repeat. If you did 5 repetitions, that would be about 45 seconds of TUT. Rather than adding weight to your lifts, think about adding tempo to your movements. Focus on the control of your movements and the tension you can create in the muscle as a way to build strength.

There are endless ways to manipulate a program, such as supersets and compound sets (to name a couple). You may have also heard of circuit training, Tabata, and HIIT training, each of which are ways to manipulate programs and get you moving. Some of these programs are designed to keep your heart rate up and to add an element of excitement during a group fitness class.

In comparison, strength training may not feel as exciting because you aren't always moving, and honestly it sometimes can be a little boring. In the beginning, it's new and different, and we use things like supersets and compound sets to add variety. The rest periods aren't very long since the weight you are lifting isn't as heavy, so you're not standing around waiting for your next set. When you start to progress in strength, the excitement comes from seeing progress over time. But during individual workouts, you are usually focused on one exercise at a time and you have longer rest periods because you are lifting heavier weight. When I first started powerlifting and training for a competition, it took me some time to get used to that style of programming. I learned to just be with myself, and to enjoy the process. Be patient with yourself during your workouts and keep your goals in mind as a way to focus your attention.

PERIODIZATION

Periodization basically means to plan or to program. There are three categories we use to create a training program. A macrocycle is a 12-month period. This is to look at the big picture: What do you want to accomplish? Do you have any competitions, races, weddings, or vacations that will impact your training? All of that should be considered within the macrocycle so that you can plan your training around them. Life always has unexpected events, but the macrocycle is there to lay out a general game plan. The second category, a mesocycle, is a phase of training within the macrocycle. Mesocycles can be as long as 12 weeks or as short as 4 weeks, depending on your goals and how your body responds to training. This is where you work to see progress from your program. For beginners, a linear periodization mesocycle focus is ideal. You would start with high volume (more repetitions) and low intensity (less weight), and slowly work toward lower volume (fewer repetitions) and higher intensity (more weight). This allows for progressive overload, which simply means adding weight or repetitions over time. Within a mesocycle, it is important not to change your

Meet Madeline

"My weight has always been a part of who I am, a defining characteristic. I was everyone's fat friend. I had a cruel childhood nickname because I was fat: 'Fatty Maddie.' And to this day, I don't really like being called Maddie. It was always to blame or not to blame for something. It was attributed to every single aspect of my life. I am a huge proponent of the body-positive and fat-positive communities. Part of this is because I was essentially 'movie bullied' as a child (and, honestly, well into adulthood). I was kicked out of my lunch table and passed notes to remind me I was fat. These aren't plot points; for some people, these are real, vivid memories. Because of that, I don't want people to experience the shame and self-loathing that I have.

I went through high school and college just fine, hating myself, but fully 'understanding' that it was fine. I had a lot of friends! I was a 'mother' to many people! So what if men were brazen enough to remind me, to my face, that they loved hooking up with me, but nobody could know they thought fat chicks were hot! I eventually learned to love myself, but that then led to a dangerous level of indulgence. I shouldn't be ashamed of who I am, so I wholly embraced it, which led to me going too far over to the other side.

When I was 27, I had a major wake-up call. I had been texting my sister about pains in my legs and kept claiming I must just be eating too much sodium. I literally had to take breaks when walking on flat surfaces. The university where I was doing grad school was at the top of a hill. It needs to be noted that, yes, this was a hill, but this wasn't a hill I dreamt about conquering. It was literally just a hill. And I was BEYOND out of breath every time I walked up it. I was always coming up with excuses to stop and trying to make it look completely normal that the fat person had to take breaks. Some people can be over 300 pounds and be completely healthy and in shape. I was not one of those people. I was putting myself into a dangerous predicament, and most importantly, I was lying to myself. I was convinced I was in fine physical shape and that body type didn't matter.

One of my roommates and I had gotten incredibly cheap tickets to go to Lithuania. I was so excited. I love Eastern Europe. It's so beautiful and I'm a sucker for beetroot ANYTHING. I'm lucky that my roommate was the person I was on the trip with because she's a kind and accepting person. She didn't miss a beat when I had to ask for a seat belt extender. I appreciate her not saying anything or trying to make the situation better or worse. Internally, I was losing my mind. I had officially hit a level where a change needed to be made. While it's true that the world does need to be more accommodating to larger bodies, I was unhealthy. I couldn't breathe, I couldn't sleep, I couldn't go on long walks. I was losing everything that made me . . . me.

I then did what everyone does when they want to make a change. I got on the elliptical for an hour straight and I hated and dreaded every second of it. For the love of God, it was BORING. But I was convinced it was what I had to do. The girl I was going to the gym with was into lifting and I started to think about how fun that would be. I had always been strong. The childhood nickname I preferred was from my family: 'Maddie Moose.' I always insisted on doing things myself. When I was three, I would insist on carrying my siblings' hockey bags and drag them across the floor myself.

I found a trainer who had similar qualifications and 'look' to my sister (who was lifting in New York and would have been a great coach, but if my sister tells me to do anything, I tend to do the exact opposite) and started. The first deadlift, I was hooked. It took focus, it took skill, and I was already kind of strong. I went all the time, loving the feeling of my muscles getting harder. I remember when my trainer gave me my first circuit and I had to do goblet squats onto a box: It felt so good to move and start feeling truly strong. I started shrinking, which was great because it allowed me some more mobility and speed in my lifts.

Flash forward a couple of years and 100 pounds lost, and I am in Brooklyn working with a different coach and doing what I said I would never do: preparing for a powerlifting competition. I have always said I wouldn't do it; I didn't want to make my happy place something that gave me anxiety. But then my mom reminded me that everything gives me anxiety, so I may as well do it. I look down at the program my coach has written me and see something jarring on it: box squats. This is something I had to do when I first started lifting because I didn't have the mobility for full squats on my own. I was now doing a different kind of box squats, one to build strength and form. I was in a completely different place. I'm still fat. I'm definitely not perfect. I fail some of my lifts and my form is definitely not always on point. But I'm a constant work in progress and what is important is that I do put in the effort and I work toward my goals. And now I'm strong as hell and getting stronger every day. I am running up hills and leaving people in my dust, I'm making gains every day, and I'm building the confidence to be the best version of myself. And I owe it all to the barbell."

Madeline

Madeline found me on Instagram and two years later she is still a client, my gym-tern, and a friend. Madeline walked in the door with big ideas about how I could make my gym a huge success. She was more than excited that I was opening a gym as a plus-size woman to create a space for plus-size women. She does a lot for me that has nothing to do with strength, but I can tell you as her coach that since she has been focused on a strength training program, her confidence and mental strength have truly grown. Madeline is a fun-loving and excited person who makes it happen. I took Madeline to her first powerlifting meet as her coach. She didn't win, but I couldn't have been prouder of her. She crushed all her workouts and showed up to the meet ready to compete. I know she was nervous, but she put herself in an uncomfortable situation and left stronger than ever.

exercise choice too much. Like we have talked about before, the only way to get better at something is with practice and repetition, so stick to similar movements so that you can create patterns and progress through repetitions, sets, and weights within your mesocycle. For example, I have a 12-week mesocycle with a focus on building the strength around my conventional deadlift. I stick with the conventional deadlift for that mesocycle and movements that help build that pattern and strength. I don't want to toggle back and forth between conventional deadlift, hex bar deadlift, and sumo deadlift all within one mesocycle, unless there is a reason to put all three in the training program.

Last, you have a microcycle, which is a week of training. Within a week of training, we want to make sure that we hit all the necessary components: an even distribution of movements, the overall volume that you are lifting, and rest and recovery days. There are seven days in a week, and most beginner programs call for lifting three or four days a week. No matter how many days you pick, you want to have days of rest and recovery between lifting days. For example, a three-day-a-week program can be as simple as Monday, Wednesday, and Friday lifting days. When you have a three-day-a-week program, there's a light, a medium, and a heavier day. For a four-day-a-week program, you have two training days back-to-back. All that means is that you should pay attention to what you are programming on those days. It's okay to do full-body back-to-back, but within a full-body program, I can split up what is being worked. For example, maybe I have a back- and quads-focused day and I have a chest- and hamstrings-focused day. The sample programs in chapter 7 give you examples.

When I first started training for a corporate company, the company wanted a program from a year out, from the macrocycle all the way through to the microcycle. I never understood why I had to spend so much time doing this, especially when every time I had a plan for my clients, something needed to change. So, here's a little secret that most coaches and educators don't tell you: It's okay to make changes. The macrocycle needs to be a guideline; it should have goals and a plan to reach those goals. Your mesocycle is a guideline for what you will be working toward and focused on within that time frame. Your microcycle is week to week. Within the meso- and microcycle, it is okay to make changes. Things happen, and life gets in the way. Write out your plan, because having guidance and a plan to reach your goals is important. At the same time, things don't always go according to plan. Expect to make adjustments as needed.

HOW MUCH SHOULD I LIFT?

You might see strength training programs using percentages of weight lifted. The idea is that you should be able to lift X amount of weight based off your one-repetition max (1RM). When you first start strength training, you have no business attempting to test your one-repetition max.

There are other ways to figure out how much to lift. Two great tools to use are repetitions in reserve (RIR) and rating of perceived exertion (RPE). Both methods take time to get used to, and I want to point out again that you should always start with less weight than you think and work your way up.

RIR simply means that you should have gas left in the tank at the end of a set; use a weight that you could lift a few more times but reserves your strength for the next set or exercise. Remember, we aren't looking to burn out and we definitely aren't always looking to hit the failure level at which you can't do another repetition. At first, you estimate to figure out your RIR, and that's okay. For example, if my program calls for 10 repetitions, I should use a weight that lets me feel like I could do more repetitions after 10. When writing a program, you could describe it as 3x10 with 2 RIR (3 sets of 10 repetitions, with 2 repetitions in reserve).

Rating of perceived exertion, or RPE, is a scale or rating based on how hard you are working. In other words, on a scale of 1 to 10, how hard is it, with 1 being easy and 10 really hard? RPE gives you the opportunity to gauge how you feel about a movement and the weight being used. You could write this as 3x10 at 8 RPE (3 sets of 10 repetitions at an 8 rating of perceived exertion), which means it should feel hard but not impossible. Generally, when we lift, we want to be between 6 and 8 on the RPE scale. If you start at or do workouts that are always above an 8, you will burn out. Aim for gradual progress. These estimations help you learn to lift smartly. Remember to start lighter than you think you need to, keep track of what you lift, and add slowly as you go.

CONCLUSION

Ready to get into your workouts? Hopefully by now you have a goal, you understand how to come up with a plan, and you understand that there are lots of ways to reach your goals. Chapter 7 gives you several sample workouts as examples of how to write a workout program. If you are new, be sure to keep it simple; don't overthink creating your workout plan. We went through a lot of information. Start simple; do what you feel confident and comfortable with. Remember not to make too many changes at once; give your body and mind time to adapt. The good news is that no matter what you create, it's hard to go wrong. Try to stick with a program for at least one mesocycle (4-12 weeks) and see what results you get. Progress isn't always about strength gains. Maybe you are moving better, maybe you feel more comfortable with the program, or maybe you stuck to something and feel incredibly proud about that.

SAMPLE WORKOUTS

Here we go, it's time for the workout! The first thing to remember is to enjoy the process, to enjoy the fact that you get to work out, not that you have to work out. Movement is a beautiful thing—it is what gets us through life. When movement is hard, it's never as hard as life can be. I like to remind myself, when I'm not in the mood to work out or when a workout is particularly hard, that I've been through worse and that people go through worse every single day. I tell myself that I can handle it, to breathe and take it one repetition and one step at a time.

In this chapter, I will show you how to write a program based on the rules we talked about in chapter 6. I will show you several examples of workouts ranging from beginner to advanced, as well as workouts that use only one piece of equipment.

Writing a workout can seem daunting and tedious, but movement is movement. A squat is a squat, and there are variations of the squat. You want to master the basics and stick with them for a while. Start easier than you think you need to, and give yourself time to progress in your program. Not all programs look the same. I broke these programs down into similar styles because it is

Checklist for Creating Your Plan

1. Determine your goal.
2. Decide how often to train.
3. Choose a type of program based on 1 and 2.
4. Pick your exercises based on 1 and 2.
5. Set your repetitions and sets based on 2.
6. Choose your weights (start light and work your way up).
7. Execute your plan and go with the flow.

easy to follow. Your workouts could have 4 movements or 10 movements; you can add tempo, RPE, and RIR; you can add assigned weights or percentages of weight. But the most important thing is to listen to your body, which tells you if you can handle more or less.

Since this book is about strength training, you won't see cardio exercises in these programs. If strength training or even working out in general is a new journey for you, I highly recommend focusing on strength first and adding cardio later. Adding too many things to your life at once leads to failure or injury. Wanting to make change and to get healthy and strong is amazing, but take it one step at a time. And don't forget that when doing a strength-based program, you are still working on your cardiovascular health. I always recommend that you spend time walking or on a bike, some type of low-impact movement. Jumping up and down is hard on the body, and it's even harder on a bigger body. Getting stronger makes all forms of cardio easier, so focus on the strength first.

An easy way to write a program is to make sure that you hit all seven of the primary movement patterns: push, pull, hinge, squat, lunge, walk, and rotate. You could do each movement pattern within one workout or spread it out over a week. It depends on how you want to do it.

Group Fitness Classes

Group fitness is amazing for a lot of reasons and works well for many people, but it may not allow you to tailor the workout to your abilities or preferences. In a group fitness class, one instructor gives instruction to a class full of students, and yet no two people are the same. Because of the limitations of the format and time allotted for the class, instructors probably don't have the time (or may not have the training and expertise) to give instructions for variations of movements as the class is happening. So, what if the instructor says, "Next, we're going to do a burpee" and you can't do a burpee? There is nothing wrong with the fact that this advanced move is not something you're ready for; you haven't yet mastered the movement pieces of a burpee such as a squat and a push-up. One of the main reasons I'm a personal trainer is because I enjoy teaching people how to do movements that are specifically right for them at that moment. If you take the time to get strong and proficient in the basic movement patterns, everything else falls into place and you'll progress to those advanced movements.

If you decide to do all seven movement patterns within one workout, you already have seven exercises for that day. You obviously don't have to do that; a workout doesn't even have to have seven movements, it could be fewer than that. Maybe between a warm-up, workout, and cool down you rack up seven, but a workout can have as many movements as you want. If you choose to split up the seven movement patterns, you do want to try and hit them all within the week. If you recall from chapter 6, I mentioned how and why we would choose a certain number of days to train and how to split them up.

The workouts in tables 7.1, 7.2, and 7.3 all include seven movement patterns in each workout. This is a three-day-a-week, full-body program, without details such as repetitions, sets, and rest. I did this because I want you to focus on the idea that every movement has a variation. There are three options for each day—beginner, intermediate, and advanced versions—to show you that every movement has a progression and regression. Not everyone is at the same point in their journey. Do the movement that feels and works best for you that day.

A note about these workouts: Just because I paired these variations together doesn't mean you have to. Not everyone is at the same level in her progression, so you can always mix and match what is best for you. You have options, and not everything has to be hard. Remember that focus, form, and tempo can make a movement plenty hard, and therefore there is no reason to only progress with weight or variation.

Table 7.1   Full-Body Workout, Day 1

	BEGINNER		
	Exercise	**Photo**	**Page**
1	Bodyweight box squat		41
2	Hands elevated push-up		73
3	Kettlebell deadlift off a block		49
4	Standing cable machine row		82
5	Step down		67
6	Farmer's carry		122
7	Pallof press		115

	Exercise	Photo	Page
1	Squat		39
2	Kneeling push-up		74
3	Kettlebell deadlift from the floor		50
4	Standing single-arm row		84
5	Split squat		60
6	Front rack farmer's carry		125
7	Half kneeling woodchop		119

(continued)

Table 7.1 Full-Body Workout, Day 1 *(continued)*

	ADVANCED		
	Exercise	Photo	Page
1	Goblet squat		43
2	Push-up		71
3	Kettlebell suitcase deadlift		52
4	Barbell bent-over row (pronated or supinated)		90
5	Backward lunge		61
6	Single-arm farmer's carry		124
7	Split stance woodchop		120

Table 7.2   Full-Body Workout, Day 2

	BEGINNER		
	Exercise	**Photo**	**Page**
1	Front rack squat		44
2	Dumbbell floor chest press		78
3	Single-arm kettlebell deadlift		51
4	Seated lat pull-down		93
5	Step-up		64
6	Farmer's carry		122
7	Kneeling plank		110

(continued)

Table 7.2 Full-Body Workout, Day 2 *(continued)*

	INTERMEDIATE		
	Exercise	**Photo**	**Page**
1	Single-arm front rack squat (kettlebell)		45
2	Dumbbell chest press on a ball		79
3	Staggered stance deadlift		53
4	Straight-arm pull-down		95
5	Dumbbell step-up (low box)		66
6	Front rack farmer's carry		125
7	Forearm plank		111

ADVANCED			
	Exercise	**Photo**	**Page**
1	Barbell squat		46
2	Barbell bench press		81
3	Single-leg deadlift		54
4	Dumbbell pull-over		96
5	Dumbbell step-up (higher box)		66
6	Single-arm farmer's carry		124
7	Plank		107

Table 7.3   Full-Body Workout, Day 3

	BEGINNER		
	Exercise	**Photo**	**Page**
1	Sumo deadlift (kettlebell)		57
2	Dumbbell chest fly (floor)		80
3	Backward lunge		61
4	Front raise		103
5	Single-arm bent-over row (dumbbell)		89
6	Woodchop		118
7	Kneeling side plank		114

	INTERMEDIATE		
	Exercise	**Photo**	**Page**
1	Hex bar deadlift		55
2	Dumbbell chest fly (bench)		80
3	Forward lunge		62
4	Lateral raise		102
5	Three-point stance single-arm row (dumbbell)		87
6	Half kneeling woodchop		119
7	Side plank (either kneeling or forearm)		113-114

(continued)

Table 7.3 Full-Body Workout, Day 3 *(continued)*

	Exercise	Photo	Page
ADVANCED			
1	Deadlift		47
2	Dumbbell chest fly on a ball		80
3	Lateral lunge		63
4	Bent-over reverse fly (dumbbell)		92
5	Dual bent-over row		88
6	Split stance woodchop		120
7	Forearm side plank		113

Now let's look at a program that uses only one piece of equipment (tables 7.4-7.6). Many of us don't have access to gyms. Or you may not want to enter a gym to work out—and there's nothing wrong with that. Remember that when building strength specifically, you do need to make sure that, over time, you are progressively overloading. Working out from home can be difficult if you don't have any equipment. However, if you are looking for a place to start, you don't need much. Plenty of people invest in home equipment because that is what works best for them. Regardless of the equipment you use, there are ways to progress workouts before you need to increase the weight.

Here is a three-day-a-week workout plan that requires only dumbbells or kettlebells. It is a full-body plan and helps you build strength. This workout is written to be done in supersets. Each exercise is labeled with a number and A or B. You do a set of A and B exercises for each number back-to-back, rest after each pair, and then do another set of A and B until you have completed the number of sets for that pair. You then move on to the next set of A and B exercises. For example:

- Do exercise 1A for 8 repetitions and do exercise 1B for 8 repetitions; that's one superset.
- Rest, then do the remaining number of supersets of this pair of exercises, resting between each set.
- Then move to superset 2A and 2B, and so on.

Notice that there are ranges within the repetitions, sets, and rest. This is done very purposely. Remember how we talked about setting a plan, but life can throw us curveballs? In an ideal world, the program would progress in a linear fashion. Let's use front rack squat as an example.

Week 1: 10 repetitions, 2 sets, rest 2 minutes

Week 2: 12 repetitions, 2 sets, rest 2 minutes

Week 3: 12 repetitions, 2 sets, rest 1 minute

Week 4: 10 repetitions, 3 sets, rest 2 minutes

What you are seeing is that from week to week, we can increasingly progress through the program, manipulating repetitions, sets, and rest. And, if you do this and feel great after every workout session and life is going well in general, you might be able to do this consistently. Let me remind you, that isn't always how life works. In the beginning of a fitness journey, you see progress happen fast and come easier to you than for someone who has been lifting for a long time. In order for you to continue to perform at your peak, you need to pay attention to how much sleep you get, the quality of your nutrition, the amount of fluid you take in, the amount of overall stress you experience, and much more. It's okay to give yourself some leeway and forgiveness in your workouts. Having ranges of repetitions, sets, and rest allows you to stay within working numbers that are beneficial to you and also gives you the opportunity to listen to your body and truly do what feels right for you on that day.

Table 7.4 Full-Body Dumbbell- or Kettlebell-Only Workout, Day 1

	Exercise	Photo	Reps	Sets	Rest	Page
1A	Front rack squat		8-10	2-4	1-2 min	44
1B	Dumbbell pull-over		8-10	2-4	1-2 min	96
2A	Split squat		8-10 each leg	2-4	1-2 min	60
2B	Military (wide) shoulder press		8-10	2-4	1-2 min	99
3A	Lateral raise		8-10	2-4	1-2 min	102
3B	Plank		20-30 sec	2-4	1-2 min	107

Table 7.5 Full-Body Dumbbell- or Kettlebell-Only Workout, Day 2

	Exercise	Photo	Reps	Sets	Rest	Page
1A	Chest press		10-12	2-4	1-2 min	76
1B	Dumbbell step-up		10-12 each leg	2-4	1-2 min	66
2A	Dual bent-over row		10-12	2-4	1-2 min	88
2B	Lateral lunge		10-12 each leg	2-4	1-2 min	63
3A	Front raise		10-12	2-4	1-2 min	103
3B	Overhead farmer's carry		30-40 ft	2-4	1-2 min	126

Table 7.6 Full-Body Dumbbell- or Kettlebell-Only Workout, Day 3

	Exercise	Photo	Reps	Sets	Rest	Page
1A	Dumbbell suitcase deadlift		6-8	2-4	1-2 min	52
1B	Dumbbell chest fly (bench)		10-12	2-4	1-2 min	80
2A	Staggered stance deadlift		8-10 each leg	2-4	1-2 min	53
2B	Bent-over reverse fly		10-12	2-4	1-2 min	92
3A	Side plank (either kneeling or forearm)		20-30 sec each side	2-4	1-2 min	113-114
3B	Farmer's carry		50-60 ft	2-4	1-2 min	122

Let's take a peek at a more advanced workout (tables 7.7-7.10). This is a general strength program with an emphasis on lower-body strength because, if you remember from earlier chapters, my favorite lift is the squat. This program has a little bit of everything and will definitely improve your general strength. You may want to customize it to meet your specific strength goals.

Notice that day 2 has a bit more of an emphasis on upper body and day 3 has a bit more of an emphasis on lower body. Remember, if you do a four-day-a-week training plan, you always have two days that are back-to-back. However, days 2 and 3 don't have to be back-to-back because you will also notice that day 3 is a heavier lifting day, which just means more load on the body. So, day 4 becomes a bit more of an accessory day and allows you to make a decision about which days are best for you to perform back-to-back.

I added a few warm-ups before each day's training, and you can obviously add more movements to your warm-ups. In the day 1 program, I specifically want to warm up the hips to make sure the glutes are warm and engaged and to make sure that the hips are ready for squats. You might add some upper-body warm-ups if the muscles in your chest feel tight that day. It depends on what your body needs and what movements are programmed for that day.

Table 7.7 Advanced Workout, Day 1

	Exercise	Photo	Reps	Sets	Rest	Page
Warm-up	Bird dog		10 each side	2	30 sec	140
	Spider lunge		5-8 each leg	2	30 sec	141
	Bridge		10-15	2	30 sec	144
1	Barbell squat		6-8	3-4	2-3 min	46
2A	Barbell overhead press		6-8	3-4	2-3 min	101
2B	Backward lunge		6-8 each leg	3-4	2-3 min	61
3A	Lateral raise		10-12	3-4	30 sec	102
3B	Plank		45 sec-1 min	3-4	30 sec	107

Table 7.8   Advanced Workout, Day 2

	Exercise	Photo	Reps	Sets	Rest	Page
Warm-up	Cat–cow		5-8	2	30 sec	138
	Shoulder dislocates		5-8	2	30 sec	146
	Reverse crunch		10-12	2	30 sec	145
1	Barbell bench press		6-8	3-4	2-3 min	81
2A	Step-up		8-10 each leg	3	1-2 min	64
2B	Dual bent-over row		8-10	3	1-2 min	88
3A	Dumbbell pull-over		8-10	3	1-2 min	96
3B	Pallof press		8-10 each side	3	1-2 min	115

175

Table 7.9 Advanced Workout, Day 3

	Exercise	Photo	Reps	Sets	Rest	Page
Warm-up	Cat–cow		5-10	2	30 sec	138
	Quadruped thoracic rotation		5 each side	2	30 sec	142
	Bridge		10-15	2	30 sec	144
1	Deadlift		4-6	5-6	3-4 min	47
2A	Push-up		10-12	3	1-2 min	71
2B	Single-leg deadlift		10-12 each leg	3	1-2 min	54
3A	Straight-arm pull-down		10-12	3	1-2 min	95
3B	Forearm plank		45 sec-1 min	3	1-2 min	111

Table 7.10 Advanced Workout, Day 4

	Exercise	Photo	Reps	Sets	Rest	Page
Warm-up	Bird dog		10-12 each side	2	30 sec	140
	Spider lunge		8-10 each leg	2	30 sec	141
	Shoulder dislo-cates		10	2	30 sec	146
1	Front rack squat		8-10	3-4	2-3 min	44
2A	Barbell bent-over row (pronated or supinated)		8-10	3-4	2-3 min	90
2B	Single-arm farmer's carry		50-75 ft each side	3-4	2-3 min	124
3A	Cable rotation		10-12 each side	3	1-2 min	127
3B	Lateral raise		10-12	3	1-2 min	102

CONCLUSION

Writing a program can seem overwhelming. But it can also be overwhelming to go to the gym or a workout without a plan. A plan keeps us consistent, and a plan helps get the job done. A training program is like a checklist. You start your workout with a list of things you want to get done and one by one you check it off. Just like in real life, with any checklist there will be changes or obstacles that get in the way of us accomplishing everything on our list. And just like real life, that's okay. But checklists and workout plans help keep us on track. They help us reach our goals. Once I've checked everything off the list, I feel incredibly accomplished.

CHAPTER 8

TAKE ACTION

What do you do once you have all the tools to start you on your path? You just start. It's okay if you don't get it right every time, it's okay to make mistakes, skip a day, miss a rep. Strength training is a part of life, and life doesn't always go according to plan. Be kind to yourself and remember that perfection isn't the goal. Progress is. A training program and setting a goal are the key to consistency, but if we don't allow for mistakes and changes, we set ourselves up for failure. This is a marathon, not a sprint. It's so easy to forget that we all fall into the trap from time to time of expecting results right away. When you are feeling frustrated or discouraged, take a breath, and bring yourself back to your mantra. As a reminder, my mindset is that I can get through anything I put my mind to. It's okay if it's hard. Do one rep at a time.

We live in a world where everything is fast, and everything is easy to find. Strength, though, takes time to build both mentally and physically. That is why strength training is so amazing. There are so many layers to it. I truly believe that people who are involved in the world of strength training understand each other a bit differently than other people do. I don't mean this in a bad way. It's about dedication. It's about wanting to work through the tough stuff, wanting to push our bodies and minds into uncomfortable situations.

This obviously doesn't pertain only to strength training. I bring this up because the difference is that people in the world of strength choose to do it. *Choose* is the key word: We choose to be uncomfortable, to sweat, to wake up at 5 a.m., and to grunt and groan. There is always a love–hate relationship within fitness, and it's okay to grunt through every workout, but remember you choose to be there, and so something in you enjoys it and wants it. It will be hard; I don't want to sugarcoat this and lead you to believe that it will be an easy journey, because it won't. But if you can bring a positive mindset and come with a plan in place, you can and will get through it.

I want to talk to my fellow plus-size women, my fellow big girls. No matter what size you are, we all got to the bodies we are in now on different paths. Some of us were born big, some of us have yo-yoed in weight, and some of us gained weight as adults. But we are all currently women in bigger bodies. We need to stick together, to respect each other and ourselves. Sometimes we dwell on the past, comparing the bodies we have now to what we used to have. "Used to" can be one of the most harmful phrases we ever use. Talking about and harping on the past won't help you make change in the now.

Meet Lynn

"I am someone who has been overweight since the age of five. I always wanted to be active and I felt like I had a lot of energy and stamina. But I was terrified that my body wouldn't be able to handle physical activity—or even worse, that people would see me and laugh. In my head, I am an athlete, but my outsides don't match—not only what others think of as athletic, but also what I think of as athletic.

Before strength training with Morit, the longest exercise program I ever maintained was back in elementary school when I did Jane Fonda's Workout record in a class after school with our gym teacher. One reason I did it was that my gym teacher didn't like me because I was fat. So I thought this would show her that I wasn't lazy and that I had commitment and follow-through. I found I actually enjoyed it; moving my body felt good and I loved the music and the camaraderie of the class. I kept it up for a couple months until the class ended, and then I was once again at a loss.

When I started working with Morit, I was legitimately petrified. I was 45 and a successful nonprofit executive and terrified by exercise—really, terrified of my body and that it wouldn't be able to do anything. I've now been working out with Morit for a year and a half. She's inspired me to be more active than I have in my entire life, to take risks, and to believe my body can do things.

Strength training has really helped me in unseen ways. My doctor commented that my metabolic rate, long way below average due to years of yo-yo dieting and hypothyroidism and anemia, had risen to a strong average level. He credits that solely to muscle mass that I've been building through strength training. I've seen positive exercise results from the inside out.

I was laid off after nearly 14 years in a job I found rewarding. It was shocking in some ways, but, in truth, it was time for me to move on. What was most shocking to me is that my CEO let me know at 4 p.m. and I had a training session with Morit at 5 p.m. There was no question I was keeping that appointment—so unlike how I had led my life before training, when I looked for every chance to avoid exercise and activity. Now, here I was with a real excuse that would be understood and instead my thought was, 'Skipping training isn't going to help this problem; sitting and wallowing won't help me.' But what did help me, and what helped me through six months of job searching, was finding strength in the routine of training—proving to myself that my body, mind, and spirit were strong. It was tough to afford training during those months. Honestly, it's still tough even in a new role. Since I'm working for a nonprofit, I don't have the kind of job that supports unnecessary expenses. But training has become so important to me that it's a no-brainer. For years, I neglected my body. Despite my treatment of it, it took good care of me. My body can do anything I need it to do, and training helps me show it the love it deserves."

Lynn

Lynn has the most positive attitude and is one of the most hardworking people I know. I hope that you were able to pick up on her determination and commitment to habit. If you could take any lesson away from Lynn, it would be that we can make excuses for anything and everything, but if you are determined and committed, you will see progress from within.

If you are reading this book, it doesn't mean that you hate being plus-size. Being plus-size can mean different things to different women. The common goal, I hope, is that we each love ourselves and the skin that we are in and that we are healthy. We should never judge each other. If a plus-size woman wants to lose weight, she should; if she wants to lift weights and get strong, she should; if she wants to remain plus-size, she should. None of these goals negate each other. I personally believe we all should love the skin that we live in, no matter the size, but if you have a goal, you should go for it and not worry about what anyone else thinks. It is the only body you will ever have; love it and treat it with respect.

Being big doesn't mean unhealthy and being small doesn't mean healthy. Unhealthy is unhealthy, and we get to decide how we take care of our vessel; no one else gets to make that decision for us. Take the time to recognize this: It's your body, your decision, and your life.

I can't bring this up enough, that the hardest part is getting started. My hope is that this book has helped you in some way. You may have learned that you are not alone, that you now have a better understanding of strength training, and that you feel good about coming up with a plan of action to get started.

Knowing you aren't alone is incredibly important. Make time to talk to friends or find people on the Internet who have the same interest in building strength. I have a private Facebook group that people join to chat about where they are in their journey. All sorts of obstacles get discussed—motivations, movements. The people in the group are there to support each other.

Some people are scared to enter a gym or work out at all for fear of being judged. Judgment comes from numerous places, such as a lack of communication, decisions made for us, and insecurities. In fitness specifically, communication is key. Often, when a plus-size woman wants to start working out, people assume it's because she wants to lose weight and they make decisions for her. It's already decided what your goals are and that there is only one way to fix "the problem." If you find yourself in this situation, communicate. Speak up for what you actually want; say so if you aren't being listened to.

I know that it isn't always easy to speak up for ourselves (I get it), but try to make sure that your voice is heard. If you join a gym, speak up. If you want to work with a trainer, speak up. If a gym isn't the right fit for you, don't give up. There are lots of gyms. It's kind of like dating: We shouldn't settle on a gym because it's convenient, and we shouldn't settle on a trainer because we are scared to break up. Find the right fit. Being comfortable with where you work out and not feeling judged are keys to your success. Remember that part of working on strength is also working on mental strength. Speaking up for yourself, your goals, and your needs is a huge part of that. Like I talked about regarding finding the workouts and movements you love, if you join a gym or are working with a trainer you don't like, you won't go; you will cancel. All of this gets in the way of your enjoyment and gets in the way of creating that habit and consistency.

It's easy to let the negative voices make decisions for us. It's easy to let other people's comments and judgments determine how we live our lives. The people who matter most won't judge us. We need to remember that there are others like us who are going through the same thing. The more we show up, the more normal it becomes to see a big, beautiful, plus-size woman lifting and doing her thing.

With 67 percent of U.S. women being considered plus-size, we are a community—we are the majority. We need to stand out more, work harder to stick up for ourselves, and normalize our bodies in all realms of health and fitness. Can you imagine when you were younger, opening up a fitness magazine and seeing a curvy woman showing you how to do a push-up? You just didn't see that in the past. Imagine how you would have felt if images like what you see in this book were also what you saw in fitness magazines or in workout videos as you were growing up. We know that our weight doesn't determine our ability, so why shouldn't we see a plus-size woman showing up and doing everything that a straight-size woman can do? What might that have changed for you if you saw that when you were younger? For me, it may have meant that I didn't spend so much of my life worrying about trying to look like the model or like my peers. I would have realized sooner that I was capable of living life just the way I was and been happy.

Showing up for yourself today makes a difference for the bodies of tomorrow. When we push ourselves and are uncomfortable today, we get to work toward our own future and the future of all the other bodies that are born different. We must set an example: Be ourselves, love our bodies, and support and respect others. By doing this, the younger generations may not have to go through the same struggle as we did.

If I could comfort my younger self, I'd remind her that my self-worth had nothing to do with my weight, that I was normal and that I should love and enjoy life. I wouldn't want her to spend so much energy and time between the ages of 8 and 27 on losing weight to fit in. Imagine your kids' futures—what do you want for them? To constantly be worried about not being worthy because of weight, or to be good people doing amazing things? We are all capable of the incredible; we can't waste all our energy and focus on something that society determined for us. The moment I figured this out, my life changed, and incredible things started to happen. One of them was writing this book!

Before you can work toward the future, you strong and confident woman, be sure to let go of the past. Many of us have yo-yo dieted and perhaps succeeded in reaching a lower weight. If you've done that, maybe you have it in your mind that you should always be at a certain weight. I advise you to consider the source of that mindset and whether it's holding you back from achieving strength goals or other positive things in your life.

Remember that some weight gain as we get older is normal. The average adult gains one or two pounds per year, so it's not likely that you will weigh the same at age 41 as you did at 21. But besides that, we have to stop living in the past; we can't keep comparing ourselves to our past selves in terms of both how much we weigh and how active we are. I hear clients say things like, "I used to be able to do pull-ups" or "I used to be able to run three miles." If your goal is to be able to do those things again, we can make that happen, but we probably won't take the same road to get there this time. Were you able to run three miles when you were in high school with not a care in the world? What does life look like now? Life is always changing, and so will the plan and the goal. If we can remember to be kind to ourselves and keep in mind an overall goal of longevity and happiness, we have a shot at being successful.

As I'm writing this book, it is 2020. We are in the middle of a pandemic, and no one could have predicted this. If you aren't familiar with what happened in March of 2020, specifically in New York where I live, everything shut down. This included my business, which also was my gym, so it was a double whammy. I bring this up because everything suddenly changed. We are creatures of habit, and when the pandemic hit, our routines were suddenly gone. Some people stopped working out altogether, while others did what they could with what they had available. After six months of gyms being closed in New York, it would be incredibly unrealistic for people to walk back into the gym and be able to do what they did back in March. This applies to anyone who has taken time away from something that they used to be able to do. If it's been a while since you worked out, ease into it. Instead of this being a negative, turn it into a positive. It can truly be a humbling experience to work hard at something again, realizing your capabilities. Know that you can do it again. Look at this as an opportunity to grow and do better. It can be a blessing in disguise, if you don't let it discourage you. If you have done it once, you have it in you to do it again, but without comparison.

Fitness truly can be a very intimidating thing—especially weights, and maybe that's why people shy away from strength training. I obviously can't stand next to all of you on this journey, but I do hope that this book helps you feel a little bit more comfortable trying. Even with all the pictures and descriptions of each movement, form doesn't come naturally to everyone. The best piece of advice I can give you is to listen to your body. When your body hurts, try to figure out if it is a hard exercise or are you actually hurting yourself? Something can be hard, but it's very different from something hurting. So, if you feel unsafe or in pain, stop. Don't risk the injury. Try changing something simple in your position, or find someone to help you. Lifting and fitness can be an individual sport, and sometimes that's what we are looking for. No pressure, no expectations, but sometimes asking for help and being around people doing the same thing can make all the difference in the world for your success.

If you were to walk away with anything from reading this book, I want you to feel confident in your decision to start a journey. There will be highs and lows, and they can be very high and very low. The wins, the personal records, the accomplishments, and the good lifts will be and feel amazing. Sometimes when we don't win all the time, that can take us down a dark path. Look at this strength journey as a marathon, not a sprint. Celebrate the small things, and don't always expect big change. Be proud when you don't let the lows take over. It wouldn't be a journey if everything always went according to plan and you accomplished everything you ever wanted without putting in the effort. Embrace the journey. Do it for yourself and no one else. Drink lots of water, eat food to fuel your body and your training, and be kind to yourself. Oh, and don't forget to squat!

ABOUT THE AUTHOR

Morit Summers has been a personal trainer since 2007, defying industry standards with her abilities and inclusive approach. She holds a bachelor of science degree in exercise science and kinesiology along with many certifications, including NSCA-CPT and CrossFit Level 1. Summers began her career at the State University of New York at Cortland. At Equinox Fitness, she progressed to a Tier 3+ trainer and began teaching classes of new personal trainers.

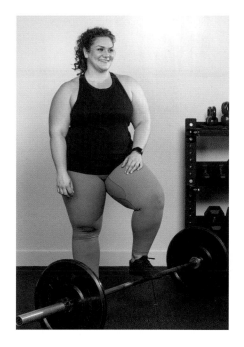

In 2016, she launched her own business: Morit Summers Personal Training. She is also co-owner of FORM Fitness Brooklyn. Clients range from individuals just beginning their fitness journeys to seasoned athletes. Aside from personal training, she is an expert fitness consultant. She has been featured in *Shape* and *Health* magazines and on LiveStrong.com; the *Good Day New York* TV show; and various health and fitness podcasts and campaigns, including Lane Bryant's LIVI Moves and Calia by Carrie Underwood's #StayThePath.

You read the book—now complete the companion CE exam to earn continuing education credit!

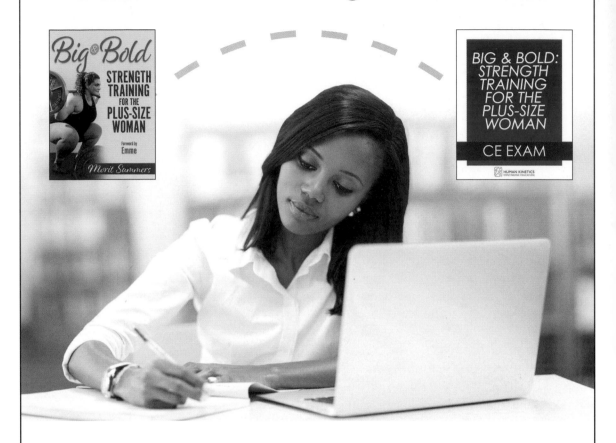

Find and purchase the companion CE exam here:
US.HumanKinetics.com/collections/CE-Exam
Canada.HumanKinetics.com/collections/CE-Exam

50% off the companion CE exam with this code

BBST2022

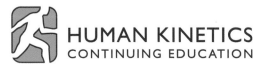